Fanning the
Female
Flame

FANNING THE
FEMALE
FLAME

HOW TO INCREASE
YOUR SEXUAL DESIRE
(WITHOUT CHANGING PARTNERS)

SUSAN KAY PRESLAR, MS FNP-C

Fanning the Female Flame: How to Increase Your Sexual Desire
(Without Changing Partners)
Published by Third Star Press
Ashland, OR

Library of Congress Control Number: 2016919749

Preslar, Susan K., Author
Fanning the Female Flame: How to Increase Your Sexual Desire
(Without changing partners)

ISBN: 978-0-9984219-0-2

SELF-HELP / Sexual Instruction

QUANTITY PURCHASES: Schools, companies, professional groups,
clubs, and other organizations may qualify for special terms when
ordering quantities of this title. For information, email susan.k.preslar@
gmail.com

THIRD ST★R
PRESS

Table of Contents

Fanning the Flame

I coasted downhill fast and liked it. Exhilarated, I welcomed the coolness on my cheeks and forehead. A car passed me on my right side. It gained momentum as we both sped farther down. The car moved in front of me and I could see it was signaling a left turn. It was braking. I saw the street that it was headed for and shock penetrated my system. The street was only a few feet ahead of me, fifteen feet at most. The car was in the left lane and turning directly into me. Impact was inevitable. I slammed the pedals back.

I was aware of the car moving on my right and the pressure of my feet against the pedals. Everything suddenly started to happen slowly as if time had become elongated and motion was suspended in something. The space around me felt oddly infinite. I felt as if I had become panoramic. I could see on both sides of me, in the front, and I could also see behind me. I could see behind me as if I had eyes on my back. I could see in all these directions at the same time. The car turned slowly into me as if it was weighted with time. It hit my front wheel and knocked the bike and me over onto the curb.

I crashed onto the cement. The slow motion suspension was over. I got up from the concrete and my body hurt— my elbow, knee, and hip hurt. The bike was torqued and the front fender twisted. I got up and walked. I walked past the café where I worked. I walked four more blocks to the three-story row house I shared with five other study-abroad college students.

The next morning I lay on a faded, purple, velour sofa in the tiny downstairs common room. It was the only sofa in the house. Jack, Ginny, Dianne, Bonnie, and Ron were still expressing concern and bringing me cups of tea. I kept thinking about the accident and how the most remarkable thing was how the moment got elongated, and how slow everything had become. I marveled that I'd seen in all directions at once, even behind me. I liked that experience a lot. I still treasure those moments and it is more than thirty years later.

Experiences that are a bit more than ordinary fascinate me. That is why I paid so much attention when women disclosed to me that they were having special experiences in their sex lives and in their relationships. Their sexual moments had become more profound, more connected, and more alive. They joined with their partners in ways that were exquisite for them and described moments of melting, merging, and feeling oneness. These women had done more than solve their vaginal dryness, or learn how to orgasm, they had found an inner "Yes!" for sex. For some, this change in their sex lives re-kindled and expanded the relationship they had with their mates. Their relationships had become more compelling. They didn't just feel mated, they felt they were in a big love affair, the love affair they realized they had been hungry for all along but had not imagined was possible. This delighted them. The aesthetic enjoyment they felt just being physically close with their partner, even when they were not having sex, was unexpected and surprisingly satisfying. Their relationships and their sex had new dimensions that were exciting, expansive, and unusually pleasing.

Personally, these stories delighted me. I liked the idea of long-term, committed couples in big love affairs, and sexual relationships that had x-factors of specialness. As a women's sexual health practitioner the stories were professionally meaningful. Women finding their desire for sex increasing is significant in this field. Low desire is the biggest sexual complaint women have. This is a fact that holds true whether you live in the United States, Brazil, Mexico, Canada, Italy, Japan, Korea, Kenya, or any other country. It is global. Low libido affects ten to forty percent of all women, which means as many as four out of ten women have low or no desire for sex. Ten percent of these women are bothered by their lack of sexual desire.[1]

Since 2002 I'd worked with this ten percent doing medical evaluations. Women who didn't feel a strong desire for sex, yet wanted to; women who missed that feeling, that interest, that urge; and women who wanted to want sex. I helped them find their desire again, or if they have never had it, I helped them locate it for the first time.

As I worked with women and listened to their bedroom stories, their successes continued to stand out to me. Women who had had no desire were finding it—even after decades of trouble with sex. Inspired, I decided to collect the stories of women who said they had successfully turned their sex lives around. In May of 2009, I did my first interview. At first I interviewed women who were either mated or unmated. I later decided to focus only on women in committed relationships. So many women came in to the office asking about their low desire while simultaneously saying they loved, respected, and were attracted to their mates. They did not want to change partners; they wanted to know how to bring the spice back into a relationship that they valued. I listened to their stories and then

1. J.L. Shifren et al., "Sexual Problems and Distress in United States Women: Prevalence and Correlates," *Obstetrics & Gynecology* 112, no. 5 (2008): 970-978, doi: 10.1097/AOG.0b013e3181898cdb.

re-listened with specific attention to the actions they took and what they saw as their turning points and insights.

If you are a woman who yearns for more satisfaction and fulfillment in the bedroom, this book is written for you. I know you can have more. Even after years of sexual unhappiness or boredom, you can move to a radically more exciting place. I am not talking about perfection or a la-la land fantasy life; I am talking about real people having an interesting and compelling love life. If you have a partner whom you respect and whom you like, and you are willing to take action and perhaps a risk or two, you already have the essential ingredients. You don't have to wait for your partner to do anything, you don't have to lose twenty pounds, you don't have to wait for the children to grow up and leave home. I promise that you can change things starting today. Instead of describing your sex life as okay or boring or painful, you can be smiling from the core of your being. You can be a woman who treasures her sexual relationship with her partner and anticipates sex with enthusiasm. You can be pleased with a capital P!

Born in the Midwest with an education that began in a Catholic grade school, helping women enjoy sex was not on my potential careers list. I studied Sociology as an undergrad, and received a B.A. from Kirkland College (now Hamilton College) in Clinton, NY. I then obtained a Master's Degree in Nursing, which was issued jointly from New York Medical College in Valhalla, NY and Pace University in Pleasantville, NY. My internship as a Family Nurse Practitioner was done at Harvard Community Health Plan in Cambridge, MA.

Before I began a practice in this sexual specialty, I was an Associate Professor at Southern Oregon University in Ashland, OR. There I was the Assistant Director, and later the Director, of the Health and Wellness Center on campus. Gynecology and sexuality were a significant part of my Nurse Practitioner practice during those fourteen years. Students came in to the health center with sexual complaints and concerns. I also led campus outreach and educational programs doing residence hall talks, sexuality fairs, and classroom lectures. I was a liaison to the LGBT club. I did more teaching and counseling about contraceptives, safe sex, sexual identity, and preventing date rape than helping women in the areas of arousal, orgasm, and desire. It was at the university, helping students disentangle the reasons for their sexual distress, that I discovered my own curiosity around sexuality. Not only was I curious about what was getting in their way; I surprised myself how strongly I lined up to help them figure it out. A bigger part of myself became engaged as their sex sleuth. I have been helping women figure it out ever since.

I chose to enter the Sexual Medicine field as an area of specialty in 2001. I resigned as Director. In the months it took to find my replacement, I continued my exploration of sexuality and began a transcontinental search for experts in the Female Sexual Health field. I traveled from Boston to Los Angeles and multiple points in between, doing internships, attending conferences, and joining professional organizations to learn more about female sexual health, hormones, and gender.

I found many *pearls*, innovative views of how to navigate some of the common obstacles women experience with sex. I was impressed by how much information and support was available to help women enjoy a better sex life, and yet, I was disheartened that these pearls were not more accessible to the public. In November 2003 I taught my first evening series for women called *In the Bedroom*. I included two other sexuality experts.

This book reveals many of the pearls I have collected, both in my quest and in my practice. I've included the stories of real women (whose names I've changed to protect their privacy) who have found their enthusiasm for sex and now have that excitement in their voices and the blush on their cheeks, which they lacked before. Each of these women had specific hurdles they overcame. I chose these women because these challenges are the ones I see most. Perhaps you will recognize some of them.

What Is This Flame of Desire?

Sexual Desire is you wanting to be sexually intimate. It is you feeling an urge to have sex. You are thinking about sex, planning for sex, and anticipating sex. There can be hundreds of different reasons why you want to have sex and the bottom line is that you want it. Perhaps you want sex so you can feel the closeness of your mate's body, or you crave the physical release of an orgasm. You may want sex so that you can feel sexually desired yourself, or because you want to satisfy your partner. You may want sex so you can feel all the delicious, heightened body sensations that come with arousal and orgasm. Your reasons for wanting to have sex will fluctuate, and so will the intensity of your desire. Sexual desire is a variable experience.

To talk further about desire we can break it into two types, spontaneous desire and responsive desire. Spontaneous desire is when you want sex without any external prompting. You are on the prowl; you feel horny. You are feeling sexual on your own, not because you are responding to your partner's advances. You are initiating the contact, making the first move, giving the first wink.

Responsive desire or receptive desire, on the other hand, is when the idea for sex originates with your partner. He or she is stroking you in the right way or whispering sweet things into your ear. They are doing something that intrigues you enough that you say yes to sex. You may experience both spontaneous and responsive desires, or just one, or you may not experience any desire at all.

One pattern of spontaneous desire is called cyclical or biological desire. Most women who are having regular periods identify this as the main way they experience their own spontaneous desire. It occurs in the middle of their menstrual cycle at the time of ovulation. You may have felt this. Somewhere between day 11 and day 16, sex is on your mind for a few days. At this time in your cycle, an estrogen surge occurs and testosterone may also increase slightly from its usual level. This is the fertile time in the menstrual cycle, so we are biologically wired to want sex during this phase.

Another time many women experience increased sexual desire is right before their period begins, and maybe the first day of the period. At this point, estrogen and progesterone are at their lowest levels of the month, and testosterone is the only hormone left standing. The presence of testosterone increases sexual desire in both men and women. Right before your period, testosterone gets to dominate the hormonal action for a day or two. This effect can increase your sexual desire (which you may like) at the same time it gives you those unwanted PMS symptoms: acne, irritability, and restless sleep (which can be annoying).

About 90 percent of the women who come to see me are looking for their spontaneous desire. They may still respond to sexual touch and they may still have orgasms, yet they miss the feeling of wanting sex without prompting. They wonder why they are no longer thinking about sex or initiating it. Where is that feeling? They want to want sex more often than they do.

YOUR DESIRE IS LINKED TO HOW AROUSED YOU GET

How excited or pleased you are when you have sex is central to how much sex you want to have. Not many people get excited for more sex if it's boring or leads to disappointment. If you want to have a high desire for sex it's important that you feel turned on and excited during sex and pleased afterwards.

Being turned on means you feel sexually aroused. Arousal happens when you respond to a sexual trigger and your body starts to get excited. Your face flushes, your breathing becomes faster, you feel hot, your nipples get erect, your vaginal walls lubricate. Your attention redirects from wherever it had been to focus on the physical sensations you are feeling.

Arousal is the signal of you saying yes to pleasure. Feeling pleasure is a good thing. The sexual pattern that women with low desire describe to me is often one of not getting aroused enough to truly get excited and feel especially good.

Sexual arousal is paradoxical. Arousal requires you to be both relaxed and excited at the same time. Your psyche needs to be relaxed enough to allow your body to build up excitement and tension for your pleasure. If you are like a lot of women, your psyche is not relaxed very often. Swirling thoughts and emotions can keep you from getting aroused even when the triggers that might excite you are present. This is common and Part 1 of the book is about this.

The best way to read this book is to remember who you are and also who you are not. You are not Snow White or Sleeping Beauty waiting to be kissed. You are not a machine looking for its missing part. You are a feminine being looking to connect sexually with enthusiasm to the one you love. You are willing to take action to make this happen.

Read this book with curiosity! You are on the hunt for your natural enthusiasm for sex. Other women have found theirs and you can too. The examples in this book are from heterosexual couples. Regardless of your sexual preference, if you are a woman this information and these strategies apply to you. Keep in mind that you are a multilayered being, you have a physical body, a mind, a certain way of moving, and an aesthetic that you project through the energy around you. These aspects of you have many variables so there is no one-size-fits-all solution.

This book is divided into three parts. Part 1 describes the mental and emotional reasons for low desire. Part 2 focuses on your body and the most common physical reasons for low desire. Part 3 lists strategies that ignite your desire. The strategies are divided into five areas of action:

- ❦ Arouse your mind and emotions.
- ❦ Optimize your body's responses.
- ❦ Empower your communication.
- ❦ Use your feminine sexuality to spice things up.
- ❦ Set the stage for delicious sexual events.

Read through the book once, and then go back and read the text boxes in Parts 2 and 3. My wish for you is that first you see how accessible a satisfying sex life is, and second that you take the action you need to find and enhance your flame.

Her breath comes into her chest quickly as his fingers land softly on the inside of her right thigh. As his warm, thick fingers trace up closer, the anticipation makes her tense, and for a suspended second her body is taut and still. Pleasure is coming. She gets it now, this cycle of pleasure. She knows she is going to yield to it and she knows it will be soon. Her mind skims through memories of last year when his touch felt all wrong. Not so now. His touch lands higher and her back begins to arch. She moves into him and kisses his neck.

PART 1

The Emotional and Mental Obstacles to Feeling Desire

In this part we are going to look at the mental and emotional obstacles that get in your way of having desire and arousal. I am not talking about ongoing anxiety or depression, which are psychological conditions that can decrease your interest in sex, but more common feelings you can experience. I have picked five that are unfriendly to your feeling pleasure in the bedroom. They are: **stress, inhibition, resentment, pressure, and boredom.**

You probably can relate to at least some of these, either in occasional moments or as longstanding patterns. I've linked each of these with a story from a woman who experienced the obstacle as a pattern and then got beyond it. I will introduce the issues here, and in Part 3 you will get to read about each woman's journey to overcoming these obstacles.

CHAPTER ONE

Stress, Sex, and the Busy Woman

Half the women I see in my office label their own daily stress level as high. Not medium, not low, but high. Life is busy, too busy. Meeting deadlines, dropping the kids off, managing the care of your aging parents, doing prep for your classes, whatever it looks like for you, you push from one thing to another.

Night after night, by the time you get into bed you are either amped up or exhausted, sometimes both. You lie there fatigued and possibly numb, not registering how soft the sheets feel against your skin, or the warmth of your partner's chest against your cheek. You are thinking about your to-do list, re-visiting something your co-worker said, or worrying about your kids. You've had so little downtime; you lie there just trying to catch up with yourself. You don't have the energy to connect with anyone else. You may not even want to roll over, let alone make love.

WHAT STRESS CAN DO TO SEX

If you are this over-busy woman, you will likely feel less desire for sex. You also will get less physically aroused when you are having sex. Research in the past two years agrees with research from the past two decades— chronic stress has a negative impact on all aspects of female sexuality. Chronic stress is defined as meeting multiple deadlines every day, something most of us do. This day-to-day stress reduces your interest in sex, your arousal, and it minimizes your capacity to orgasm.[2] It also negatively affects your general health. Stress increases cortisol levels in your blood; extra cortisol increases body fat and your risk for heart disease and diabetes. It decreases your fertility, your immunity, your thyroid function, and unsurprisingly, your appetite for sex. In addition, prolonged stress can create other hormonal changes that lead to fatigue and depression, which dampen desire.

When your own life is too busy and stressful, sex is no longer centered on your enjoyment; it becomes something for you to get through—another task to check off your to-do list.

Jane, 45 years old, had this kind of sex life with her husband of over twenty years. In their most intimate moments, her legs up in the air and breathing fast, Jane planned her business projects. Her head was filled with thoughts that had nothing to do with what was happening to her body, they were not erotic at all. Instead she was planning how she would meet her next deadline. Though her body was physically involved in sex, her mind was not.

At work, Jane was a dynamic woman with an entrepreneurial nature, yet in the bedroom she did not take any risks. Jane told me that it was the stress in her busy daily life as well as some residual negative feelings towards men that contributed to her being so cautious and reserved.

---

2. Lisa Dawn Hamilton and Cindy M. Meston, "Chronic Stress and Sexual Function in Women," The Journal of Sexual Medicine 10 (2013): 2443-2454.

As a 15-year-old high school freshman, Jane began dating a popular guy in the junior class. She felt honored that an upperclassman athlete would want to go out with her and they dated through her entire four years of high school. He pressured her to have sex right away, and she went along with it, but she did not find it enjoyable. It was never about her pleasure. Sex was all about his feelings, his pleasure, his timing. Looking back, she realized that her boyfriend's behavior had been inconsiderate at best and at worst mean, but she did not recognize it then.

At home, her father and brother frequently criticized her body. They would squeeze her butt and tell her it was too big. They pinched her breasts and told her they were too small. They said no one would ever date her with a body like hers.

Jane now sees that that kind of touching was abuse, though it was not labeled abuse back then. Her dad and mom engaged in inappropriate sexual actions in front of her and her siblings. She was mortified by their displays. These early experiences framed sex and men's sexual behavior as negatives in her mind.

When it was time to go to college, Jane took that opportunity to move as far away from her home environment as she could, relocating from upstate New York to California. Three weeks into her freshman year, she discovered she was pregnant by her high school boyfriend. Lying on the table after the abortion, she made a promise to herself: "Today is the last day I will ever make a bad decision for myself."

She then began to date "wonderful" guys. In her senior year she met Tom, and they married a year later. They soon had a daughter, then a daughter who died in infancy, and a few years later they had a son. Their family life moved along, their personal careers evolved. In the evenings after work, she earned her MBA. Jane and Tom shared parenting duties based on who could squeeze in what between work responsibilities. Things between them were fine, though their schedules stayed packed for years.

Jane describes their sex life during these years as super-basic and herself as a super-guarded woman in bed. "He'd never been with anyone else before me, so anything was great for him. As for me, I didn't have a good experience in the past, so I would say that our sex was nice but never great."

Over the years, her husband became interested in trying different things, varying sexual positions, or having sex in new locations. She was not interested. They stuck with the same two positions, and always in the bedroom. Even though at work she demonstrated bold, creative leadership, in the bedroom she stuck with the usual experiences. "Our sex life was humdrum. But for me that was fine because it was safe. We did not have discussions about what we liked, and I never thought of moving his hand to a different place."

Their relationship and sex life remained status quo until their children were both in high school. Jane then found personal time for herself, and she started doing what she called self-work. She began to exercise and lose weight. She began to feel physically strong and enjoy being in her body. As she started to like her body, she took better care of it. She felt more attractive. As Jane exercised regularly, her stress level also dropped. Jane began to activate and feel alive in a way she had not experienced before.

As Jane invested in herself and began to enjoy life more, she and Tom grew apart.

"When you add raising children plus life's busyness and stress to a boring sex life, people start looking somewhere else," Jane said. "We were bored, and we both started interacting and flirting with other people."

CHAPTER TWO

Inhibition—Not Feeling It's OK to Express Yourself

SUPPRESSED SELF-EXPRESSION

Like Jane, many women don't feel comfortable expressing themselves in bed. Even women with dynamic personalities who live colorful lives outside the bedroom tone themselves down when they are having sex. They constrict their movements, lower the volume of their voices, and limit the types of sounds they make. Sometimes this is due to feelings of shame and negativity around sex. Sometimes it is due to other factors. Suppressing your self-expression reduces your sexual arousal. Uninhibited women get more aroused and orgasm more often than women who hold back.[3]

When I started studying women and sexual desire, I was surprised at the number of forces I found that encourage women

---

3. David Farley, "The Role of Assertiveness in Female Sexuality: A Comparative Study Between Sexually Assertive and Sexually Non Assertive Women," Journal of Sex & Marital Therapy 17, no.3 (1991): 183-190.

to curb their impulses and suppress their expression in bed. I was amazed that any woman manages to be open and available sexually in the face of all of it. Let's look at some of the reasons women struggle with the inhibitions that limit their pleasure.

Body Self-Consciousness and/or Body Shame: The thoughts and feelings you have about yourself can have a huge impact on the level of sexual freedom you feel. If you are highly critical of your own body, or fear your partner's criticism, these thoughts keep you from feeling confident and freely moving your body during sex. Worrying about whether your stomach is too big, or if your breasts are too small, or if you're too fat, or not pretty enough all can keep you from wanting to be seen naked. This worry can make you less vocal and more reserved than you would be if you freed yourself of these inhibiting thoughts.

Your partner's close attention on your body may make you uncomfortable, and you may catch yourself monitoring how you look from your partner's point of view rather than relaxing into your own sensations. This self-consciousness also may have you hurry through sex. You want it to be over, so you can end the discomfort you feel about being seen. You don't express this discomfort, or frustration, or even your pleasure. You contain all your feelings and move on.

Children at Home: When the kids are home and asleep, you may keep the lid on your self-expression so you don't wake them. You also prefer to remain quiet, so you can hear them if they need something. If they are awake, you might half expect them to pop into your bedroom unannounced, so you stay on the alert and ready for that. You don't sink into your sexual experience as freely or deeply as you would if they were not there.

Under Aroused: Women who don't feel aroused enough often retreat to an inhibited, non-communicative position rather than share with their partner what is going on. You may be thinking that your arousal is taking too long or wondering if your partner is frustrated or bored. You might hesitate to admit the truth about not being turned on, or you fear if you speak up, you might find out he *is* bored (which he probably is not), so you say nothing.

Avoiding Feelings: If you have a pattern of controlling your feelings, you may have trouble allowing yourself to open up and feel them during sex, even when you're with someone who has shown you their love is tried and true, and they are not likely to judge you. You may be aware of a build up of unexpressed feelings and fear the flood that may come if you acknowledge even one of those feelings.

Guilt, Fear, or Shame about Sex: Experiencing guilt, fear, or shame while receiving pleasure can keep you from moving toward more of it. Pleasure can be linked to shame and anxiety due to prior trauma such as sexual abuse, religious conditioning, or other influences that make sexual arousal a mixed up and confusing event. You may freeze up, or push through, rather than slow down and speak up. You may have trouble finding the words to express your discomfort.

Social Conditioning: In addition to these internal forces, we live in a culture that constantly broadcasts conflicting messages about females and sexual desire. Subtly or emphatically, women are told that receptive desire is the only *good* form of sexual desire for women. It is OK for you to respond to your partner's interest in having sex with you, but it is not ladylike for you to display your own hunger for sex yourself.

As wondrous, life affirming, and wholesome as female sexuality is, there is no positive language to describe it. I have not been able to find words in English that link feminine goodness with feminine desire or feminine arousal. Even if you are in a relationship with someone you love deeply, or in a marriage of years in length, we don't yet have a word for you and your love of sex.

We do have negative words to describe women who enjoy sex and their sexuality: slut, whore, loose, easy—even if you're not aware of it, this ambiguity on a cultural level can subconsciously impact your enthusiasm for and your capacity to let go or feel sexual pleasure.

Although Jane still chose to be sexual with Tom, she did so in a partially inhibited state for years and years. It was not just the stress that decreased her enjoyment; she was self conscious and unassertive. Looking back she called herself boring and repetitive. She never felt safe enough with men to express honestly what was going on inside her body and mind. Disclosing these intimate details was not even on her list of possibilities.

Still, sex was important to her even when she was distracted by her daily stress and inhibited by her past. Jane did expand her sex life, first by focusing on herself and her body, and then by challenging the inhibitory thoughts in her head. She found out what worked for her, and you will read how she did this in Part 3.

CHAPTER THREE

Pressure-Can I Say No Again?

A big obstacle to sexual desire is feeling pressure around sex. Women of all ages come to me asking for help with handling pressure from many different sources—pressure to have an orgasm, to be a good girl, to avoid pregnancy, to try to get pregnant, and so on, but the most frequent pressure they ask about is how to deal with sex when their partner wants sex and they don't.

Sofia, age 26, called for an appointment saying she wanted to talk about her low sex drive as it was causing relationship problems. She and her 29-year-old boyfriend, Nathan, had just broken up after a big fight about sex.

Nathan asked her for sex frequently, maybe once a day or more. It felt like too much to her, and she had other things to do. She wanted to have sex; she liked sex, but not that often.

A week later Sofia drove up from her home in Northern California to see me. During the days since our initial phone call, she had relaxed some. She had read an article about libido and realized that her low sex drive was not abnormal, as she had feared. Also, she and Nathan had reconciled a few days after the break up. They had missed each other tremendously, and she said, "We are going to figure things out—especially the sex thing."

According to Sofia, honesty and being real were fundamental components of her relationship with Nathan. Together for two years, they both valued creativity and spontaneity, and to top it off, they were highly attracted to each other. Sofia was in love with Nathan and described him as handsome, creative, and fun.

She still wanted to be with him, but the sex part was hard. He wanted sex too often for her. She was afraid this difference meant they were not compatible. She hoped this was not the case.

When Sofia filled out her medical history form, it was nearly blank. There were no ongoing or past illnesses. No fatigue, no insomnia, no depression. She was not on any medications. She had no symptoms associated with hormonal issues. We did not order any hormone or other lab tests for her. She was a healthy, young woman.

During that first appointment Sofia also disclosed that she had another aspect adding to her confusion. She was born into what she called a "traditional family with traditional values."

"You are definitely told not to have sex before you are married," she said. Even though she had not adhered to her family's values around sex, she still felt stuck between the pressure of Nathan's desires, and the pressure of her family's values. None of her sexual decisions felt like her own. She found herself indecisive when Nathan wanted to have sex, and she was not sure what she wanted. She waffled in her communication with him and it added to her and their confusion.

Not long after our meeting, she was with her whole family at her sister's wedding in New Jersey. Her parents expressed their delight that her sister was a *pure bride*. This exacerbated Sofia's conflicted feelings. In the midst of her boyfriend's desire and her family's values, she was under pressure to figure out what she herself wanted.

We will pick up Sofia's story again in Chapter 3 to see how she became more confident.

CHAPTER FOUR

Resentment-When You Want to Like Sex as Much as He Does

We all feel resentment from time to time. Resentment usually means our needs or desires are not being met. Things seem unfair. When there is resentment towards your partner, even if the resentment is not about sex at all, sex can be less appealing as a result: less intimacy, less arousal, less satisfaction. In Pam's story, the resentment was specifically about sex.

"I thought my husband Luis was a good man, yet I had resentment. I resented that he got more pleasure from sex than I did. He was enthusiastic about sex, and I was not. I didn't have real issues with sex, but I had never been really into it. I'd never felt I had to have sex. Sex had always been somehow a little negative for me."

Pam, 46, came into my practice not for an issue with her sex life, but for help with her hot flashes and her moods. She had had an early menopause, before age 40, and had been taking estrogen and progesterone for the past six years to help with the symptoms. On her symptom survey on the day of her first visit, she happened to check the box for low libido. I asked her about it. Pam said things had started out OK sexually with them. But now, after twenty-nine years, even though she loved and respected her husband, Luis, when it came to sex she felt resentment.

"We got married so young, and in our early years of marriage I was so into pleasing him, it made me feel good to make him feel so good. Then things changed."

Some of the change was parenting. "My whole life revolved around my kids for so many years."

And some of it was not knowing what to do to get more aroused, "For a long time, I didn't understand why I couldn't just have an orgasm from the sex act itself, intercourse. I didn't understand why it wasn't the same for me as it was for him."

Because her sex drive was lower than her husband's, Pam thought something was wrong with her. She never asked for help because, she said, she felt embarrassed. She worked in a loan office, and she noticed the women at work talking about sex with more enthusiasm than she'd ever felt.

Pam's husband never expressed his concern about her sex drive directly. He had heard that a woman's libido peaked around age 40, and he had joked a few times that he was looking forward to their turning 40 together. When her periods stopped at 39, her desire dropped even further. That long-anticipated peak never came.

Pam continued to ignore her thoughts and questions about sex and went on with her life, not giving sex too much attention. When they had sex, it was OK, but sometimes her resentment would keep her from having an orgasm. Sometimes she would wear a flannel nightgown to bed and hope that it would decrease his interest.

As their kids got older, their son got married and their daughter moved to Arizona, Pam realized their relationship had changed without the children in the house. If she did not try to cultivate something with Luis, they would grow apart.

When I had asked Pam about her libido during that first office visit Pam realized that other women had the same problem, and her low sex drive was more common than she had thought. It was a turning point for her. She signed up for the *In The Bedroom* class for women I was offering the following month.

At first, she was not even going to tell her husband she was taking the class. She thought she would just explore and see if anything happened as a result. Pam ended up telling Luis about her plan to take the class before it started, and shared with him why she wanted to take it. In that conversation he was open and supportive. His openness and his lack of defensiveness was a relief to her.

"I kind of cracked the door open a little bit, and he was totally receptive to anything I had to say. So after that, I felt a little bit safer."

This was the beginning of Pam's exploration of her low libido, and we will find out the rest of her positive story in Part 3: Strategies for Fanning Your Flame.

CHAPTER FIVE

Boredom-When the Sexual Connection Is Not That Interesting

Have you ever thought as you were having sex, "Same old same old" or wondered, "Is this all there is? All the hoopla about having sex, and this is what they were talking about? Where is the excitement, the connection, the pizzazz?" One expert described boredom in the bedroom as this: when things you like are not happening and when what is happening you don't like. Boredom is a real experience for both women and men. The disappointment associated with boredom is quite real too. This is true even when your love and regard for your partner remains high.

Ruth always adored her husband; she respected him and was proud to be his wife. It was a confusing surprise to find out that she didn't connect with him sexually.

She met Bill when they were both in their late thirties. They each had "done work on themselves" and were in good places. Their relationship started with a close level of communication and connection and they got married a year later. He was self-employed as an electrician and was valued by people in his church and Rotary. She liked that he donated his time to local building projects and to charities.

She said she did not dread having sex, but she did not look forward to it. When he made sexual advances toward her, she felt herself shut down. She did not want to shut down, but she did.

She thought this reaction might be because as a massage therapist with almost twenty years' experience, she had developed a fine-tuned sense of touch. She knew what kind of touch she wanted on her physical body, and Bill's touch was not that. She did not know what else it could be. They had worked with a therapist, and they'd seen some success in communication, yet nothing changed in her experience of sex. They had sex about once a month.

Connecting with him outside the bedroom, but not in, was perplexing and painful. "There was not a lot of pleasure in it for me." After ten years of disappointment and confusion, Ruth came to accept that their sex life was the way it was and became resigned that it might never change. She decided that she could tolerate not having a great sex life. She was disappointed, but she was not going to leave the marriage because of it.

In Part 3, you'll get to hear how Ruth and Bill's sex life transformed.

There are four main reasons for low desire in women that are tied to hormones.

PART TWO

The Physical Obstacles to Sexual Desire

When you are on the quest for a higher libido, looking at your physical body and knowing how it works is important. In the early twentieth century and even more so before then, sexual problems in women were viewed as primarily psychological. Not so now. What is going on in your head is important, and just as vital is what is going on in your physical body. The two are inter-connected, and together they create your experience of desire.

Part 2 describes the most common physical causes of a woman's low desire for sex. This includes hormonal conditions as well as other physical influences. *Don't skip this section. Even if you are healthy and have no physical problems, read these chapters anyway. You could be surprised. It is not uncommon for a woman to have someone else point out a hormonal symptom as a symptom, while she herself had thought it was just her normal. At the least, after reading, you will appreciate your body and all the complexities in it that are working well.*

Also note: the treatments that these women used are reported in detail, including the medications they used. Their treatments are specific to them. Your care and your choices will be specific to you. You will read about things that work and get ideas, and yet these choices may not apply to you. Medications and hormones, even over-the-counter ones have risks involved. Please consult with a knowledgeable health care provider before beginning any new medication or product, even if it is sold over the counter.

CHAPTER SIX

Four Hormone-Related Causes of Low Desire

1. Hormonal Birth Control *Heather's Story*
2. Menopause *Trisha's Story*
3. Low Testosterone *Paula's Story*
4. High Testosterone (e.g., Polycystic Ovarian Syndrome) *Ann's Story*

Before we get into each one, let's take a bird's eye view of hormones and how they function. Hormones are messengers, chemicals that transport signals to your cells and cause them to change. They do far more than regulate your period or your pregnancy. Hormones affect your mood, growth, weight, hair, skin, orgasms, sense of aliveness, and your ability to concentrate. The key hormones that influence your sex life are estrogen, progesterone, DHEA, testosterone, thyroid, cortisol, and insulin.

Let's break this down some more. These hormones can be sorted into two main categories—steroid hormones and peptide hormones.

Steroid hormones influence your sexual development and

fertility. These include estrogen, progesterone, DHEA, and testosterone. Steroid hormones are made from cholesterol. After you are born your adrenal glands and/or ovaries convert cholesterol into these hormones.

Peptide hormones, such as thyroid and insulin, can affect your sex life by affecting your energy level, your sleep, your weight and/or your mood.

Too little or too much of these hormones and you will have symptoms. Genetics, the environment (both your environment now and when you were in utero), and lifestyle all play a role in your hormonal configuration. I could write an entire book on just hormones, but for our purposes here, I am going to focus on the four most common hormonal causes of low sexual desire.

HORMONAL BIRTH CONTROL

Heather was thirty-one when she first came to my office for help to locate her sexual desire. Her sandy blonde hair had an angled cut that came right below her chin. She walked in, sat down in the office chair right up against my clinic desk, and looked directly at me and said, "Tell me Susan, do women ever really want it?"

As she asked me that question, I took a quick breath as I registered what she was telling me—that she did not experience sexual desire, and that possibly she never had. Even though her particular medical situation has presented dozens upon dozens of times in my office since her visit in 2003, I will never forget the striking directness of her question.

Heather told me she'd never felt interest in being sexual. She did not think about sex or look forward to it. She never had. She otherwise had a very satisfying life. She was attracted to her husband. She found him to be exceptionally good-looking and manly.

Heather was healthy. She had no medical conditions. She was

on no other medication besides the pill. Her life was busy and she enjoyed it. Mostly she stayed home with their three school aged kids, and she assisted her husband in his CPA practice part-time. Their daughter was eleven, and their twins (a boy and a girl) were nine. All of her children were well adjusted.

Her contraceptive history revealed that she had gone on the birth control pill in her late teens before becoming sexual. She was on birth control when she married her husband, and she had stayed on birth control pills until she wanted to get pregnant. She stopped to get pregnant and then started again when she stopped breastfeeding. She did this again for the second pregnancy when she had the twins. She had gotten pregnant quickly each time. At the time of her visit she was back on the pill.

Although highly effective at preventing pregnancy, birth control pills and other hormonal contraceptives are not always sex friendly. They can dampen sexual desire and reduce vaginal lubrication during sex, which can cause intercourse to become painful.

Research shows that while most women on the pill report no change in desire, some report more sexual desire, while others report less.[4] I see those women who have less.

Here's why some women see their desire drop. Hormonal contraceptives (including the pill, the patch, and the ring) prevent pregnancy by blocking ovulation, so that surge in hormones that comes with ovulation no longer happens. If you are used to experiencing a spontaneous interest in sex mid-cycle, you may notice that it is no longer there after you start using a hormonal contraceptive.

Also, hormonal contraceptives lower the testosterone level in your body. Testosterone, which is the primary hormone associated

---

4. Laura Burrows, Maureen Basha, and Andrew Goldstein, "The Effects of Hormonal Contraceptives on Female Sexuality: A Review," The Journal of Sexual Medicine 9, no. 9 (2012): 2217.

with sexual desire in both men and women, is produced less by your ovaries when you are on hormonal contraceptives. Also, the estrogen you are taking causes a liver protein called Sex Hormone-Binding Globulin (SHBG) to be increased. This protein binds up your testosterone, making the testosterone that you do have less available for your cells to use. Lowering your testosterone can land a blow to your sexual desire. It also can decrease lubrication, sensation, arousal, and weaken orgasm—all the feel good parts of sex. The Ortho Evra Patch, the NuvaRing, and also the newer, lower, twenty microgram estrogen birth control pills create even more binding up of testosterone than the older versions of the pill that had thirty or thirty-five micrograms of estrogen.[5]

Birth control pills (rings and patches too) lower your testosterone levels; this drop in testosterone might lower your desire for sex, cause vaginal dryness and reduce the feel good qualities of sex.

Heather's blood tests confirmed her testosterone levels were below normal and she had an elevated SHBG level. I explained to Heather that this is a side effect of using the pill and it did not mean something was wrong with her.

After our visit Heather decided to try going off of the pill to see what she experienced. Nine months later, she came in and reported that she had started feeling cyclical sexual desire about seven months after stopping the pill. This pleased her. She could finally relate to *wanting it.*

She never went back on the pill. Since both she and her husband were satisfied with their three children, he got a vasectomy.

Their sex life expanded. She continued to desire him, especially mid-cycle. She discovered a newfound appetite for exploration and discovery. They got creative in their lovemaking—they were sexual

---

5. Burrows, "Effects of Hormonal," 2215.

in the middle of the day and in different rooms of the house, they bought sex toys, and experimented with anal intercourse. They became far more open with each other and felt more connected.

Heather told me feeling sexual desire has made her feel normal. She's no longer missing out! She finally felt part of the club of women who have desire and enjoy sex. She did not realize how much she had felt like an outsider before.

Some contraceptives don't block ovulation or lower testosterone; these include the barrier methods—condoms, diaphragms, and also the PARAGARD® IUD (Copper-7). There is always the vasectomy option for your partner, or a permanent method for you, if you both are sure you don't want any more children.

Not everyone is a candidate for these methods. Your medical history, your risk of pregnancy, and your personality all should be factors in your choice.

If you notice a drop in libido within a few months of starting *any* hormonal contraceptive, explore your options with your health care provider. The list of possible problem birth control methods includes the progestin only contraceptives like the Depo-Provera shot, the mini pill, and the implants in your arm, as a small percentage of women users may have lower libido and vaginal dryness with these as well. There is no perfect contraception, as each has its plusses and minuses.

If you do need contraception and your situation requires you to use a hormonal contraceptive that blocks ovulation or lowers your testosterone, there are remedies that can counterbalance those negative effects. Also, some birth control pills are found to be friendlier to your sex life than others.

MENOPAUSE

You have most likely heard a lot about menopause and sex; jokes are made about it, groans are heard, and there can be whining. The sexual changes can be significant. Menopause is not an optional event and you will go through it if you have not already. The menopausal women that I see want to have an active and great sex life with vaginal wetness, good sensation, and robust orgasms. The bad news is that the physical obstacles are real, and if you relax and let nature takes its course, your sex life will most likely be diminished. The good news is there is no better time in history to be a post-menopausal woman who wants to have a great sex life. There are many supportive actions you can take, and being proactive is a positive.

American women are now living to an average age of 84 years. The average age of menopause is 51 years. This means you will have thirty-three years after menopause to have sex. That is a third of your lifetime!

I will start with a description of menopause in general, and then I will dive into its sexual consequences. Natural menopause occurs gradually. As the number of eggs in your ovaries reduces from the two million or so you were born with to about three hundred, your ovaries stop releasing eggs. When ovulation stops, the ovaries no longer produce estrogen and progesterone. As the hormone levels decrease your period becomes irregular, and will, over a year or two, stop. This drop in hormone levels causes your symptoms.

There is no better time in history to be a postmenopausal woman who wants to have a great sex life.

Surgical menopause is when your ovaries are removed surgically, often because of a hysterectomy. This is an abrupt change in hormone levels and one can experience multiple symptoms within weeks of the operation. Naturally, you will have no more periods after this surgery.

Some women are comfortable as their periods become irregular and menopause follows, while other women become distraught with a high level of physical symptoms. Of course, symptom levels can vary in-between. Sixty percent of women see a health care provider seeking relief. The other 40% don't have symptoms, or they are not significant enough to choose medical help. Some of the common symptoms: feeling hot, hot flashes, night sweats, sleep interruptions, and/or mood changes such as irritability, anxiety, or depression.

Symptoms of Menopause

Feel hot and have hot flashes
Have night sweats
Irregular periods
Vaginal dryness
Increase in frequency of urination
Can't get to sleep and/or can't stay asleep
Mood swings and mood changes
Feel anxious
Feel irritable
Feel depressed

Menopausal symptoms are the most intense the first year after periods stop. They can continue for years, about seven-and-a-half years on average, and they do become less intense over time for many women, but not all women. 2015 research shows 42% of women who are between 60 and 65 still have moderate to severe symptoms.[6]

The two biggest menopausal obstacles that will affect your sex life are a lowering of your desire for sex, and vaginal dryness. A vital thing to know is that these sexual symptoms, the vaginal dryness

---

6. "The North American Menopause Society Statement on Continuing Use of Systemic Hormone Therapy After Age 65," Menopause 22, no.7 (2015): 693.

and the changes in libido, are not the menopausal symptoms that resolve with time. These persist for the remainder of your life, and the vaginal dryness is often progressive, unless treated. The dryness can lead to sexual pain. You will need a strategy to deal with these two changes if you want to maintain a satisfying sex life.

POST MENOPAUSAL LOSS OF LIBIDO

Hundreds of women have told me, "I love my husband, but I am no longer interested in having sex." Hundreds! Millions more are out there. More than 500 million women in the world are post-menopausal.[7] Many of these woman still *want* to be interested in sex, they just aren't.

Trisha was 62 years old when I first spoke to her about her sex life. Her drop in libido came with menopause, twelve years before. The change happened gradually, and sex with her husband became non-spontaneous and predictable—a once-a-week event, always at the same time in the same way—something like scratching a mutual itch, she said, "If we're lucky enough to have the itch." Although they'd had wonderful, compatible sex with each other for decades, it had become *"Boring,"* she said, *"and we don't do boring."*

Trisha had noticed this happening for a lot of her girlfriends—they were having less and less sex. "What I've seen with my friends is that because they've lost interest, due to menopause, they don't feel motivated. They can't see the point of revamping sexuality because from where they are, they don't want to. What's the point? They don't feel sexy, they don't feel horny, they don't need sex anymore, so what the hell is the point of exploring it?"

Trisha was looking for options. Sex had been such an important and a strong part of her relationship with Ted, and they both wanted

---

7. K. Hill, "The Demography of Menopause," Abstract. Maturitas 23, no. 2 (1996): 113-127.

the spice back. She had high regard for Ted. They had felt *chemically attracted* to each other from the time they'd first met in their twenties, and she wanted that back.

A vital thing to know about menopause is that vaginal dryness and decreased libido are not symptoms that resolve with time. They continue, and the vaginal dryness is often progressive.

Part of the boring part for Trisha was that she used to orgasm during intercourse when she was on top, but she had not been able to do that for the past several years. The only way she could *make it* (have an orgasm) was through oral sex. In the past, she had been resistant to receiving oral sex. Once she began to experiment with it, she discovered how pleasurable it is, and she began to enjoy it. Still, she missed the variety of sexual options she'd previously had.

Trisha signed up for my *In the Bedroom* class with the hope that it might help her figure out how to rekindle the spark she and Ted used to have.

When she told Ted she was going to take the class and why, it opened what she termed a scary conversation between the two about their current sex life. It was difficult and painful, but each of them found the courage and the honesty to say the hard stuff. They both admitted being bored with their whole pattern around sex. They agreed that sexuality was important to them, and that they were at a turning point. They were in their early sixties, and they both wanted to remain sexually active for another twenty or twenty-five years. Something needed to shift.

Trisha said that part of having the courage to broach this topic with Ted was she knew that they were supportive of each other. Neither was out to criticize the other. They both knew they wanted the same outcome: an exciting sex life. "It takes a lot of trust. Trust and knowing that you have faith in your partner, that you both want

Sexual pain due to lack of lubrication is preventable, and the earlier you treat the dryness the less treatment you will need.

the same thing. It's a huge, huge part of it," Trisha said.

Trisha's loss of libido was caused by a change in her physical body, and yet her solution was not a physical one. She did not take hormones. I will explain how she and her husband recaptured their spark in Part 3.

Whether your cyclical desire is gone due to surgery, menopause, or medication, there is a similar landscape to navigate. It is confusing, and can feel like a huge loss, sometimes devastating. One client, amidst tears and angry shouts, expressed how furious she was that no one had told her she would lose her mid-cycle interest in sex. She said she would have appreciated it more when she had it if she had known some day it was going to be gone.

For women in a lesbian relationship at menopause, when ovulation stops, it can be doubly confounding. This is especially true if both women stop ovulating at or around the same time. With neither partner having that spontaneous cyclical interest, sexual initiation can drop sharply.

VAGINAL DRYNESS

When women feel wet just thinking of sex, or when sexual touch sets off that arousal cascade, it is from a fluid coming through the vaginal walls and collecting in the vagina. The medical term for this process is *transudation*. I will call it arousal fluid. This fluid that comes with arousal is thin and watery, and is created, as far as we know, to facilitate sex. Armpits sweat when a woman is nervous and excited, a vagina's "sweat" happens when the woman is sexually excited. Wetness is important to a woman's sexual pleasure. It lubricates the vagina for ease of vaginal penetration and the pleasure sensations that can lead to orgasms. Women like wet sex. In a 2012 study of 2,451 women whose average age was 32, 56% said they preferred sex to be "somewhat wet" and 36% preferred it to be "very wet." That is a total of 92% of the women preferring wet sex.[8]

Your vagina is a flexible, muscular tube, lined with a membrane that has its own world of microbes and blood vessels. When estrogen declines in your whole body the decline shows up in your vaginal tissue in predictable ways, most notably dryness. Thinning of the vaginal lining creates this dryness. The vaginal lining (called epithelium) can be forty to fifty cells thick before menopause, and it can get as thin as three to seven cells thick after estrogen declines. Women who could previously enjoy twenty minutes of thrusting now feel burning pain in their vaginas after thirty seconds.

When your estrogen declines, the vaginal pH goes up, causing your vagina to lose friendly bacteria, and making you more prone to yeast and bladder infections, or symptoms that mimic those infections. Vaginal dryness is common. A 2011 study reported 56% of women between the ages of 40 and 84 reported having vaginal dryness, and 83% of those women were bothered by it.[9] Other studies publish similar or greater numbers.

Vaginal dryness occurs frequently in young women too, often associated with use of hormonal birth control, or other hormonal conditions. The most popular treatment is a low-dose, minimally absorbed estradiol cream that is applied topically around the vaginal opening and inside. Other successful treatments come in the form of vaginal rings, vaginal suppositories, and pills. The main thing to know about sexual pain due to vaginal dryness is that it is preventable. And the earlier you treat it, the shorter and less costly the treatment will be. Treating dryness right away keeps you from developing

8. K.N. Jozkowski et al., "Women's Perceptions about Lubricant Use and Vaginal Wetness During Sexual Activities," The Journal of Sexual Medicine 10, no. 2 (2013): 489.
9. R.E. Nappi and M. Kokot-Kierepa, "Vaginal Health: Insights, Views & Attitudes (VIVA) – Results from an International Survey," Climacteric 15 (2012): 36-44.

tight pelvic floor muscles, something I will say more about later in the book. If you have vaginal dryness, whether it is from hormonal contraceptives, menopause, or other hormonal imbalance, you can find fast and effective treatments, resolving dryness in as little as eight weeks.

LOW TESTOSTERONE

Testosterone is widely regarded as a male hormone as it is the dominant sex hormone in men, but you have testosterone too and you need it. Called the *horniness hormone*, testosterone drives your desire to engage in sex. It also positively supports your sensations, your arousal, and your orgasms.[10] It helps to keep your vulvar tissue strong. In your whole body testosterone brightens your mood, increases your muscle strength, your stamina, your energy, your concentration, and your optimism. I frame it as the *Energizer Bunny* hormone because it supports your action and alignment in getting things done. Yet you don't need much of it, a little goes a long way. Similar to men who have small amounts of progesterone and estrogen compared to their levels of testosterone, you have small amounts of testosterone to go with your more abundant estrogen and progesterone.

A precursor to testosterone, DHEA, is produced in the adrenal glands, and it is also referred to as a male hormone. These male hormones are normal in a female body. When you are still having monthly cycles, roughly half of your testosterone comes from your ovaries and half is converted from your adrenal glands. These hormones are referred to as androgens.

Of the low libido women who come to see me, roughly two or three out of twenty will have testosterone levels so low that I identify it as a contributing factor to their low sex drive.

---

10. Mohit Khera, "Testosterone Therapy for Female Sexual Dysfunction," *Sexual Medicine Reviews* 3 (2015): 138.

Paula was 49 years old when she came to my office with a frustration. Her sex life had changed, and she could not figure out why. She had no impulse to have sex. She was not even thinking about sex. She also said that the sensations in her vagina and clitoris had become dull. "It feels like I'm made of cardboard down there."

Her nipples being stroked or squeezed did not turn her on the way it used to. Her orgasms took longer, and felt duller or shorter than before. She described herself as feeling less alive, "I feel deadened. I don't feel like a woman."

Paula and her husband owned a dairy farm. She was up early every morning to do the daily chores that had been a part of her life for more than twenty years. When asked about muscle strength, Paula said lifting things above her head had become noticeably difficult. Overall she was weaker and less toned, even though she was using her muscles just as much. She was noticing more fatigue than usual. Before, even if she was tired, she could push herself to get something done. She could reach inside herself and find some energy. Not anymore.

Paula had always been a bright and upbeat person, but her optimism had decreased. She felt inexplicably low. She had trouble recalling names of people and places, and she would catch herself drifting off, lost in thought.

Paula was exhibiting the classic symptoms of low testosterone. Low testosterone affects your whole body, not only your sex life. When her blood was tested, it turned out all her androgen hormones were low.

As we age, testosterone levels decline as Paula's had done. The decline starts before menopause, in our thirties and forties. Chronic or acute stress, hormonal contraceptives, and daily use of narcotic pain medications can speed up the decline. Also, women who've had their ovaries removed are more at risk for low testosterone than women who still have ovaries.

Paula was prescribed a 2 mg lozenge of testosterone to take daily along with two over the counter supplements (Vitamin B complex and Ashwagandha). She was prescribed a topical cream to use vaginally that combined low dose estrogen in the form of estradiol (.1 mg/ml) and testosterone (1 mg/ml) that she applied to her vaginal area twice a week. At her eight week follow up, Paula reported feeling better in all ways. She felt more robust and optimistic. Sexually she no longer felt like she was made of cardboard. Stimulation felt arousing and enjoyable. She did not need to use a lubricant during intercourse.

Your testosterone level can lower so gradually that you might not notice the change at first. You might habituate to your lower energy levels and forget what it felt like to have had energy. Even though your fuel tank is empty, like Paula, you might keep going and doing all the tasks you did before you felt tired. Despite feeling drained you push yourself to complete your day. This fatigue and burnout will compound your low sexual desire. By the time you get in bed, there is no oomph for anything. You are wiped out. Sleep may make you feel a little less tired, but you are still low in energy when you get up in the morning.

When getting treated with testosterone replacement therapy, you only need a small dose. Men who are deficient receive 50 to 150 mg a day. Women usually need only 1 to 4 mg a day. Big difference. It is important for you to take just enough, as more is not better with its use. (Also, you don't want to be taking testosterone when you get pregnant, as it is not safe in early pregnancy.)

We do not yet have an FDA approved testosterone product for women in the US. The upshot of this is that knowledge among healthcare workers about testosterone varies widely from provider to provider. Choose a provider who is familiar with its uses for women. If you get a prescription, you will be prescribed a product that is designed for men and told to use a small percentage of a man's daily dose, or you will be prescribed a medication that is from a compounding pharmacy made specifically for you.

In the year 2000 Procter & Gamble made a daily testosterone patch of 3 mg for women. It went through the FDA review process without raising any red flags, but it was not released due to a lack of data on long-term safety. Other countries did approve it and are using it. Information is being gathered on its safety. Also, new DHEA and testosterone products for women are currently in FDA trials so there may be more options for females shortly.

Symptoms of taking too much testosterone include: intense PMS (Premenstrual Syndrome) symptoms, anger, short fuse, acne, restless sleep, sweating, anxiety, hair thinning on top of the head, extra body hair, and period problems.

Symptoms of Low Testosterone in Females

Decreased stamina

Decreased muscle formation and muscle strength (i.e., muscle weakness)

Sense of fatigue

Lowered optimism/depression

Decreased vaginal and clitoral sensation

Decreased nipple sensation

Vulvar burning, vaginal tears after intercourse

Thinning quality or lessening volume of hair on the body

Decreased desire or no desire for sex

Dullness of memory

If you have three or more of the symptoms on the list above see your health care provider for an evaluation. If your tests show that you are deficient (below normal range) or low normal (low normal is the bottom 25% of the normal range) you may be a candidate for treatment.

HIGH TESTOSTERONE

About 10% of women in the US (20% of the women I see in my practice) have a relative excess of androgen hormones or have been diagnosed with PCOS (Polycystic Ovarian Syndrome). PCOS is a genetic hormonal pattern. In PCOS, DHEA and testosterone are robustly influential in relation to your female hormones (estrogen and progesterone).

Even though testosterone is widely accepted as the hormone of desire, if you have too much, you will not necessarily have a high libido. You may still have similar desire problems, or arousal and orgasm problems, though not for the same reasons.[11] Let's back out and look at the big hormonal picture. With this hormone pattern women often experience problems with their periods—skipped periods, frequent periods, heavy bleeding, extra long periods, severe cramps, or no periods at all. Some physicians prescribe oral contraceptives to manage the pain and the bleeding, and to make the cycle regular.

Women who have heavy and/or long periods can bleed so much that they become anemic. They can become so tired from an iron deficiency that they don't have the oomph to be interested in sex. On top of that, it can seem to your partner that you are always on your period, and never available for sex. Misunderstanding around this can lead to distance and resentment in your relationship.

Even if periods are regular, with the extra androgen influence, women with PCOS are more likely to have cycles without releasing an egg. Without that mid-cycle hormone spike, they are less likely to experience the cyclical desire I wrote about earlier. Also, not ovulating means a woman is not producing much progesterone. Progesterone

---

11. L. Lara et al., "Prevalence of Sexual Complaints and Epidemiological Profile of Women with Polycystic Ovary Syndrome," The Journal of Sexual Medicine 12 (2015:12 supple 1): 61.

is the relaxing hormone in your chemical mix. You have receptor sites in your brain for progesterone and when it lands there, you can feel mild sedation and relaxation. Often, with low progesterone your sleep is restless, and you don't wake up feeling restored.

Women with high testosterone report to me having night sweats, itchy or hypersensitive skin, and greater irritability—sometimes too irritable to want to be touched. They also are more likely to be depressed.

Many women with PCOS struggle with weight. The extra androgen increases the size of your muscles, sometimes this works for you, and sometimes your muscles bulk up more than you want. This bulking up increases your weight. Excess body weight can contribute to a lack of desire for sex. Many women who gain weight become self-conscious about their weight. It inhibits them from wanting to be seen naked.

Not all women with PCOS have or are going to have all of these symptoms. Many women with PCOS have no sexual problems. There is a large variation in how women with PCOS are affected. The underlying hormonal pattern is there, but the expression is different. With genetic studies, we are still learning why this expression is so varied.

Besides low sexual arousal and desire, women with excess androgen hormones can complain of vaginal symptoms including burning, dryness, or irritation. Some women report their own lubrication does not last long enough for them to finish sex without needing to add a lubricant. Sometimes there is ongoing itching and burning of the vagina that gets worse at certain times of the month.

Ann had this PCOS hormonal pattern. It was her anxiety and irritability that brought her in for a hormone evaluation. Specifically, it was the flush of embarrassment on her twelve-year-old daughter's face when she, Ann, angrily demanded that the ice cream man turn down the annoying music coming from his truck. She recognized that her reaction was over the top and she was tired of being on the edge. On her intake form, Ann marked her symptoms—anxiety, irritability, vaginal dryness, specifically vaginal burning after intercourse, low libido, restless sleep, and worsening PMS. She had felt on edge for a few years and the number of days she felt moody was on the increase. Her sexual desire had been low for years. The vaginal dryness had started after the birth of her second child and was getting worse. Lubricants helped intercourse feel comfortable, but she was not that excited about having intercourse at all. She had sex because she knew it was important to her marriage, and she did like the closeness she and her husband shared after sex.

The vaginal dryness and burning that is sometimes found in women with PCOS is easily treated. Ann found this to be true. Eight weeks after she began treatment, her vagina felt back to the way it was before she had her second child. She no longer had dryness, and she no longer burned for a few days after being sexual. These vaginal symptoms responded quickly to the same estrogen treatment used for menopausal vaginal dryness that I mentioned earlier: a topical low dose estradiol cream, or suppository used once a week.

Ann was placed on a prescription of micronized progesterone, and she felt more relaxed and was able to sleep longer and deeper. She no longer experienced on the edge, moody feelings. She still felt anxious at times, but the feeling was slight in comparison. Her husband could approach her without her snapping at him. His touch, which had become annoying, felt good again. Intercourse was distress free, and she felt stronger levels of arousal than she had in years.

Heavy Periods

Periods can be heavy for a number of reasons, including hormone imbalances. When periods have heavy flow or last for many days watch out for anemia. Iron deficiency anemia is common in women with heavy periods. Anemia will make you tired and low in mood. Heavy bleeding is defined as a need to change your pad or tampon every one to two hours. Long periods are defined as longer than seven days. If you become anemic, treat the low iron until your hemoglobin and hematocrit are in the normal ranges. Usually the treatment is increasing iron in your diet along with over-the-counter iron supplements. Sometimes prescription iron is recommended. Also, if your provider doesn't test your ferritin level (a measurement of stored iron), ask for it. Clinically, I notice women with ferritin levels greater than 50 report a stronger sense of well being and are more likely to have some energy left for sex when they get into bed, than women with ferritin levels below 50.

One in ten women have PCOS. Your lifestyle, diet and hormonal management are all factors in managing this genetic hand you have been dealt. You can play your cards in a way to feel your best sexually, as well as to balance your mood and energy.

Also, your health care provider can help you look at several treatment options to help you modify the heavy bleeding. Some of your options are friendlier to your arousal and libido than others. When your hormones are managed well, you will have more regular cycles, and probably lighter periods. You will discover you have more choices around which days to be sexual, and more energy with which to have it.

Having PCOS is like being dealt a hand of genetic cards. You can play those cards so that you feel your best, sexually and in terms of energy and mood. Your lifestyle, diet, and hormonal management all are important pieces to managing the hand you were dealt. Remember you are not alone; one in ten women has a similar set of playing cards.

Here's a list of the most common symptoms with this hormonal pattern:

Symptoms of Too Much Testosterone in Females

Acne
Restless sleep/Insomnia
Irritability
Anxiety
Short fuse/Anger/Rage
Worse PMS
Menstrual Cramps
Weight gain/Bulking up
Irregular periods/No periods/Heavy periods
Facial hair and excessive hair elsewhere on body
Thinning scalp hair on top of the head
Vaginal irritation and/or dryness

CHAPTER SEVEN

Other Physical Obstacles

SEXUAL PAIN

Mindi remembered the thrill and enthusiasm she felt when she and her husband Tim were first dating. She was eager, and so was he. They did not have intercourse before they got married. They did other enjoyable sexual things and her body responded with excitement. Both of them looked forward to going all the way. After they got married, though, her excitement level changed. The thrill and enthusiasm disappeared. She was not sure what happened, the only thing she came up with was maybe it was a mental switch. Mindi said, "I just lost what I had."

On top of not being interested, later in that first year sex became painful. She felt a stabbing pain at the beginning of intercourse, and sometimes deep penetration caused intense pain. Mindi was not wet enough inside, and even though she and Tim used lubricants, it was not enough to keep intercourse from hurting.

Mindi still wanted to be sexual with Tim, and like many women with sexual pain, she opted to go ahead and have sex anyway. Even though she was in pain nearly every time, Mindi tolerated this for years.

During the first years of the marriage, every now and then, when, as she and Tim joked, "the stars and the planets and the moon and the sun aligned correctly," and she was in the mood and sex was not as painful, she had some good experiences, but she couldn't say why. Maybe it was her hormones, maybe it was because she'd had a sexual dream or saw a romantic movie. She didn't know. Those events weren't frequent enough to allow her to figure it out.

Mindi had started on birth control pills one month before she got married. We now know that birth control pills can cause a lack of lubrication and pain with intercourse in up to 10% of young users;[12] this knowledge wasn't available at the time Mindi started taking the pill. She had only stayed on the pill for a little over one year, yet the cycle of sexual pain that lack of lubrication can cause had been triggered.

Pain during intercourse can lead to a secondary problem: tight pelvic floor muscles. This was true for Mindi. With painful intercourse, a woman will reflexively grip her pelvic floor muscles. The muscles stay tight and they get shorter. This creates muscles that sit higher than they used to when they were relaxed. These elevated muscles are tender, and have sensitive trigger points. When the thrusting of intercourse hits these elevated tender muscles, it hurts. It may leave insides feeling tender or bruised for days after sex.

Even anticipating sex that hurts can cause the muscles around the vagina to tighten. Shorter pelvic floor muscles can make the vaginal opening smaller and tighter, so that any kind of sexual penetration becomes difficult or highly uncomfortable. This bracing grip may

---

12 C. Bouchard et al., "Use of Oral Contraceptive Pills and Vulvar Vestibulitis: A Case-Control Study," American Journal of Epidemiology 156 (2002): 254-261.

continue during intercourse too—a far cry from what women want to experience in the bedroom.

After more than sixteen years of suffering, Mindi sought treatment for both the vaginal dryness and the subsequent pelvic floor pain. Mindi had never forgotten the level of sexual excitement she'd first experienced. It had become a marker for her of what was possible for her to feel. She wanted to get back to that. At her first exam I referred her for pelvic floor physical therapy, and started her on the vaginal estrogen cream. She saw the therapist about eight times. She was given homework to relax her muscles when she was by herself, as well as relaxation exercises to do during sex. As her muscles relaxed, both the pain at penetration at the vaginal opening and the pain deeper inside lessened.

Mindi used the topical estrogen cream twice a week for a few months and then dropped to the maintenance dose of once a week, and then stopped using it. If she were still on the pill she would most likely need to continue the vaginal estrogen once a week or so until she stopped taking the pill. Mindi did get back to the enthusiasm she had first experienced about "going all the way." Treating her dryness and getting rid of the sexual pain was her essential first step.

If your pelvic floor muscles become too tight you need to work with a physical therapist who specializes in pelvic floor work. Some talented instructors who teach core strengthening or Pilates understand the pelvic floor too. Left untreated, a pelvic floor muscle spasm can go on to cause hip and low back pain. It also affects urination, as too much or too little tone contributes to leaking urine when you cough or sneeze.

Although it requires investing some time and money to have the treatment sessions, it's well worth it. Many women get better after eight to ten physical therapy visits. If you continue to do the exercises at home, not only can you get rid of pain and problems with bladder control, you can improve your sexual responses. Relaxed pelvic floor

Intercourse should not hurt. If you have pain, don't live with it, seek an answer and keep talking to your health care provider until you are pain free.

muscles allow for more blood flow, and more blood flow means more arousal, and more arousal means more pleasure and more orgasms. Having a relaxed yet toned pelvic floor is important if you want to optimize your sexual experience.

Vaginal dryness, whether as a side effect of birth control or from menopause or PCOS, is the most common reason for painful intercourse that I treat in my practice. There are multiple other reasons for painful intercourse. If you have pain with intercourse don't live with it, seek an answer. Some pain is just at the vaginal opening, and other women have pain deep inside. None of this pain is normal for you to have. Intercourse should not hurt. Sex should not be painful unless you have mutually consented to an S & M activity. Talk to your health care provider, and keep talking until you have an answer that resolves the pain.

FATIGUE

If night after night you get in bed so exhausted that the pillow is more attractive than the man or woman in bed with you, it may be time to figure out why you're so tired and make some changes. After all, you can't have a great sex life if you come to bed tired all the time.

Common Reasons for Fatigue:
- Not enough sleep
- Low iron (especially in menstruating women)
- Low thyroid
- Low testosterone
- Depression
- Chronic Stress

If you think your fatigue is due to lack of sleep, leave more time for sleep and see if your fatigue resolves. For optimal health and sex drive most women need seven to nine hours of good sleep a night. If you are already sleeping eight to ten hours and are not feeling refreshed when you wake up, see your health care provider and ask to be evaluated for fatigue as something else may be going on. Sleep should be restorative. If you leave time for sleep and can't get to sleep, then your insomnia needs to be evaluated.

Fatigue and libido are not good bedmates; if you want to increase your sexual desire, figuring out why you are tired is part of that package.

If you know it is your lifestyle that doesn't allow you to get to bed before you're wiped out, be aggressive in changing your lifestyle. Go to bed earlier. If you can't because there is just no way in your life to do it, and nighttime does not work for you, find a time of day when you do have energy for sex. Morning? A lunch date?

Fatigue and libido are not good bedmates, so if you want to increase your desire for sex, looking at your fatigue is part of that package.

MEDICATION

Check your medications and over-the-counter products to see if you are taking something that is known to decrease your arousal, desire, or orgasm.

Here's a list of the most frequent offenders:
- Antihistamines
- Progesterone
- Oral estrogen
- Anti-depressants

- Hormonal birth control
- Benzodiazepines
- Opioid pain medications
- Blood pressure and heart medications

If you are on something that is not sex friendly see if there is something else you can take instead. You might be able to change the medication, change the dose, or add something new. There is often something you can change to counter the negative effect. For example, oral estrogen, which binds up testosterone, can be changed to a transdermal (through the skin) option such as a patch or gel. That change alone can free up more testosterone to be available in your body. If you have the vaginal dryness associated with use of birth control pills, a weekly application of low-dose, minimally absorbed estradiol vaginal cream can take the dryness away. If you are on progesterone for the night sweats and insomnia associated with menopause, or to decrease your heavy periods, you can get a side effect of sedation. This is convenient for helping you sleep at night, yet if the dose is too high for you, the sedation can make you feel so relaxed that you feel limp. It is hard to get sexually excited when you are too relaxed. Lowering your progesterone dose may be a possibility.

Anti-depressants are the biggest cause of sexual side effects in women in the US today. Eighty-five percent of the prescriptions used to treat depression in the US are in the group with known sexual side effects, SSRIs and to a lesser degree, SNRIs. Even if you're not on one of these drugs, you've probably heard of them: Selective Serotonin Reuptake Inhibitors (SSRIs, brand names Paxil, Prozac, Zoloft, Celexa, and Lexapro) and Serotonin Norepinephrine Reuptake Inhibitor (SNRIs, brand names Cymbalta and Effexor) can disrupt your desire for sex, decrease arousal, and interrupt orgasms.

If your sex life has worsened since starting one of these medications, discuss the changes with your healthcare provider. Be specific about the symptoms. Your provider may be able to switch an SSRI anti-depressant to an SNRI (less disrupting), or to a dopamine/norepinephrine (Wellbutrin) prescription that may be less disruptive or possibly supportive of your desire. Or they may add another prescription, such as taking Viagra, which has recently been shown to be helpful to women achieving orgasms while on anti-depressants.[13] Also, there is data from Australia that shows the use of testosterone can increase the number of "satisfying sexual events" you can have when on anti-depressants.[14] Or you can try a natural solution, such as adding aerobic exercise. Aerobic exercise prior to sexual stimulation was shown in a 2011 study to increase the sexual arousal in women on both SSRIs and SNRIs.[15]

Another natural way is to increase the time you and your partner spend arousing you. Know that your medication makes it harder to get excited, so give your body more attention and more time to get there.

If you checked in with your provider three years ago about your anti-depressant side effects impacting your sex life and you didn't get helpful answers, check in again. There are new medications on the market that are more sex-friendly and one may be appropriate for you. Be persistent. Not all providers take your sex life as seriously as you would like them to.

13. H. G. Nurnberg et al., "Sildenafil Treatment of Women with Antidepressant-Associated Sexual Dysfunction: A Randomized Control Trial," The Journal of the American Medical Association 300 (2008): 395-404.
14. E. Fooladi et al., "Testosterone Improves Antidepressant-Emergent Loss of Libido in Women: Findings from a Randomized, Doublie-Blind, Placebo-Controlled Trial," The Journal of Sexual Medicine 11, no. 3 (2014): 837.
15. T. A. Lorenz and C. M. Meston, "Acute Exercise Improves Physical Sexual Arousal in Women Taking Antidepressants," The Annals of Behavior Medicine 43, no. 3 (2012): 352-361.

PART THREE

Strategies for Fanning Your Flame

Y ou have come to the fun and juicy part of this book. You now get to read how the women in Part 1 connected with their sexual pleasure. What did they do to get there? This section includes a list of strategies, and woven into these strategies are the "how they did it" parts to their stories.

The strategies are all action items and most you can do immediately. No more waiting for life to hand you your libido back, and no more waiting for your partner to get things going for you. These actions are unilaterally yours. You are the one on the move and you are the change agent.

I've divided these strategies into five action areas:

- 🌹 Arouse your mind and emotions.
- 🌹 Optimize your body's responses.
- 🌹 Empower your communication.
- 🌹 Use your femininity to spice things up.
- 🌹 Set the stage for delicious sexual events.

CHAPTER EIGHT

Arouse Your Mind and Emotions

REMIND YOURSELF "I DIDN'T PROMISE TO BE PERFECT."

"I didn't promise to be perfect, I promised to show up." This is the mantra to repeat to yourself if your own thoughts and emotions get in your way of a great sex life. If you get stalled out by thinking you are not good enough or pretty enough, that you don't like your body, or you need to lose thirty pounds first, remember this: you are not promising perfection, you are promising to be close and sexual with your partner.

Our minds can be over active. Thoughts that do not support having a great sex life can parade out one after another. When women don't enjoy sex they often think there is something wrong with them. I hear this a lot. Chances are that you are fine sexually. There is nothing wrong with you. The main thing you need to do is interrupt the negative thoughts that stop you from moving toward sexual intimacy. Inhibit the thoughts that inhibit you. Encourage the thoughts that bring you closer.

You don't need to lose weight to connect or have an orgasm. You don't need to have a perfect body. You don't need to be in the perfect mood either. You can show up for sex feeling awkward. You can feel shy, resistant, or confused. No matter what you're feeling, if you want to have sex, you can still choose to have sex and enjoy it. You don't need to be a perfect anything to enjoy sex. Remember you are not promising to be perfect and neither is your mate. You are promising to show up and connect.

Let's go back and revisit Jane, a dynamic and creative business-woman who was restrained and "boring" in bed. When we left her story in Part 1, Jane and her husband were drifting apart. They were not connecting sexually, and they were flirting with other people.

Jane did not have an affair, but Tom did.

At first Jane was devastated. She told him she wanted a divorce. He was clear he wanted to stay together.

Remember, you are not promising to be perfect in bed and neither is your mate. You are promising to show up and connect

During their big "divorce conversation," they agreed to hold off for six months before they made any decisions about whether or not they would separate. They agreed to "lay low" and "keep talking."

Jane said, "I started examining my own issues that were so defeatist toward men and myself. I had never been okay with myself. I realized that I had never had good sex. After all those years, going all the way back to age fifteen, I had never worked through my feelings about men. I discovered that my underlying opinion about men was that they were scum. Even though I didn't really believe that, I think that voice just kept going on and on and on in my head. That thinking comes out in really bad ways in my relationship with my husband—even though my relationship with my husband had been really positive."

Jane realized that many things she had been doing in her work life were attempts to mask how she felt inside. She would take on huge tasks and major projects, just trying to prove to herself that she was okay. She would pile on more and more and then "conquer it."

She used her work as an excuse to keep her mind so busy during sex that she didn't have to be present and intimate with her husband. On a subconscious level, she believed if she were busy enough, she wouldn't have to feel her old childhood feelings of shame and anger. The biggest turning point that Jane identified was reframing her view of men. She did this with the help of a psychotherapist, and also a shaman. As that changed, she and her husband began to connect with greater intimacy.

"Just listening to each other and talking about what feels good and what doesn't feel good, telling him to do *that* more, made a difference. Before, I would never have reached out and moved his hand so that it felt better to me. Little things like that started making a difference in us being more comfortable together."

She kept working out, getting her body in shape while she was also working on the inside on her attitude about herself and about men. As she felt better and better about her body, it translated into better sex with her husband. She was more comfortable being seen naked, which she found was important and helped her feel more confident as she began to communicate what she liked in bed.

"I let myself get more in touch with my feminine, and that has been, I have to say, an absolute blast. I wear pretty nighties to bed, and Victoria's Secret lingerie. I now wear pink for the first time in my life. I visualize myself as a lady, a pretty lady. I know this sounds strange, but having a strong role in business and having to perform at high levels in intense meetings and negotiations, it has been difficult for me to turn on the feminine. It's like I just forgot how to do it. So concentrating on letting myself be a lady is an exciting challenge and actually kind of empowering—not to mention my husband eats it up!

After the divorce conversation Tom kicked it into gear. He made changes too. He began taking the lead in some of the decision making for the first time in twenty-three years. I liked that he was stronger and not so reliant on me. He basically got his ass in gear. My respect for him grew, and that had a great deal to do with me enjoying sex and love with him more."

Jane likes herself more now. She accepts herself. "Overall I feel like a better person, a more generous person." Jane's thoughts are about having fun as a female, and sometimes that means thinking about and doing erotic things. She thinks about sex ahead of time, and contemplates what she would enjoy. She expresses herself. Her daring and creative aspects have made their way into her sex life.

Work plans still try to crowd into her thoughts during sex, but she experiences the pleasure and enjoyment more. She has experimented with different ways to be sexual with her husband, different acts, positions, and places, and she is asking specifically for the things that please her. Her desire for sex has increased, and she is enthusiastic about their relationship.

Her enthusiasm for the relationship is made up of many personal moments. Sometimes, she says, Tom anticipates what she needs before she even realizes she needs anything, and the surprise in that delights her. He also relates to her more personally and on a moment-to-moment basis, which brings about a closeness that feels good. Often they find themselves on the same page about a choice before they even talk about it. "It is as if I am in a big love affair, the kind I hoped for but didn't think was possible."

If you keep thinking that you want a more exciting sex life, yet you never take an action to change anything, examine your thoughts. Are you repeating certain notions that take you away from wanting to be sexual? Do your thoughts encourage you to postpone taking action? Do you have ongoing self-critical thoughts? If so, get help. See a counselor. Jane did and it worked for her. Remember: you did not promise to be perfect, you promised to show up.

Be Honest about Your Internal Experience

When you are in the bedroom (or wherever you are having sex) it pays to be honest about what is going on inside of you. Is your mind spinning out in a world of its own? Are you uptight? Pissed off? Inhibited? Bored?

Let's say you are in bed, it is 10:30 pm, and your partner has let you know that they are interested in sex. You have mixed feelings. You want to be fully aroused and into it, but you are not. You may feel resistant or vulnerable, yet you still would like to be sexual. You are trying to decide whether to go with the suggestion or not. You are getting an internal YES and a NO at the same time. It is confusing. You want to shift to a full green light and go for it, but you don't know what to shift.

If you have mixed feelings like this, your partner can play a big role in getting you to a YES place, and that can be a *good* thing. Take a risk and disclose what is going on inside you. Give him or her a chance to meet you where you are. If you disclose that you are feeling vulnerable, he may say he likes shy women. If you cannot get your mind away from the office, he may say I bet I can help you do that. He is not talking you out of the way you feel, or convincing you to have sex that you don't want, he is working with you and the complexity of your feelings. You are a woman who wants to have a great sexual encounter, and in the moment you don't have an internal green light, yet you want to have one. Being honest with your thoughts and feelings can contribute to your finding one. You both want to have great sex; you are both on the same team in making great sex happen.

Let's go back to Pam's story. As you may recall, Pam struggled with resentment. She felt sex had always been somehow a bit negative. She did not get into it all that much, and she resented her husband because for him, sex was really enjoyable. When we left her story in Part 1, Pam had just told her husband she was going to take my class. He had reacted to that news with support.

"I kind of cracked the door open a little bit and he was totally receptive to anything I had to say. So after that I felt a little bit safer," Pam said.

Later, Pam took another leap and disclosed her resentment. She told Luis that she had resented him for years because he enjoyed sex more than she did. When she revealed this, he remained relaxed and supportive, and was not defensive. He said he would be willing to do anything she needed to help her. His open and supportive stance, Pam said, created a safe space for her to explore herself. She identified this as a turning point for them.

"After I got over the part where I resented him, I was open to any suggestions he had. We tried different things, and sex became more exciting for me. I made suggestions too and we experimented with different ways to arouse me. I found that lovemaking with long, slow strokes and few words turned me on more, so we did that. I pleasured myself in front of him. It wasn't about trying to masturbate; it was a joint thing with my husband. I showed him what gets me aroused. He got pleasure out of it. When I'm happy and pleased, it's better for him. Doing that did not make him feel less masculine.

I learned a lot more about myself sexually. I had to get over the awkwardness of talking about sex and not be so weird about it. When I got over that, our communication was better."

"I had to get over the awkwardness of talking about sex and not be so weird about it. When I got over that, our communication was better."

Pam's honesty with Luis about what was going on internally with her led to a string of good changes in her sex life. Sex is way more positive for her now. She can now completely give herself to Luis, and she could not do that before. This new level of sexual connection has made everything in their relationship more positive. It has filtered through their whole life and marriage. Not only does Pam like sex, but she enjoys just being around Luis, and they understand each other better. She enjoys being with him even if they are at the hardware store together. For years she said she did not realize how important sexual connection was to their overall connection. Now she sees what a huge part it plays.

In talking together about sex Pam learned that Luis had been thinking that she did not find him attractive because she did not initiate sex. This was not true. She definitely found him attractive, but she had not figured out how to make sex work for her. Her lack of initiating had nothing to do with how attractive he was to her.

In her exploration to find a way that she liked to orgasm, she said she got relief from the pressure of believing that there was some right way to have sex. She absorbed the point that there isn't something wrong with her, or with him, if she does not orgasm from intercourse. She found a freedom in the bedroom that she had not had before.

For years she did not realize how important sexual connection was to their overall connection. Now she sees what a huge part it plays.

Pam said her favorite thing so far is when her husband met her at the door with a drink, drew her a bath, made dinner, and after dinner placed a sexy lingerie outfit on the bed. She says what increases her interest are all the little things that he does for her that say he cares. (These things increase her responsive desire!). She now is more honest and direct about what all those little things are.

PAUSE YOUR BUSY THOUGHTS AND FOCUS ON YOUR SENSATIONS

As a capable woman accustomed to getting things done, often by using your mind, it can be frustrating when things work differently in the bedroom. Many women with high levels of responsibility struggle to shut down their internal dialogue. Their attention doesn't become absorbed in the sex that they are having because it is busy elsewhere. It's wonderful to be a goal oriented, successful woman, and yet when you approach sex that way you are missing the point. Sex is not about getting the job done or doing things right. It's about being present, in the here and now. So forget about getting somewhere. It's not about you *DOING* anything (for once), but rather an opportunity for you to feel, not to do. So allow yourself to feel your sensations, and let pleasure take you to new places.

When you are having sex, pause your busy thoughts. Take your attention away from the non-sexual thoughts and focus your attention on what you are physically feeling. You will have far more exciting and captivating sex if you do this. It may not be easy to keep your attention on your sensations, but it is worth the effort. Even if your body is joined with your partner's, if your mental focus is miles away from the action, sensations of heightened arousal, merging, timelessness, and synchronicity won't happen. Magical moments occur when both your body and mind are present.

When you're having trouble leaving your mundane thoughts behind, the only item on your to-do list is to take your attention away from those thoughts. Take your attention and put it where the action is. Put it inside your vagina and on your clitoris. Put it on your skin and on your breasts. If you find it wandering away from the action, invite or pull it back to your body again. Think of your attention as a thing that you can move around and then move it. You will immediately feel more arousal or sexual tension when you do this. It is surprising how quickly your arousal will increase when your attention is on the sensations you are feeling and not with your circling thoughts.

If you can use more support to keep your attention on your body's sensations, you may download my audio exercise and use that to help change your attention habit. It is available on the website www.fanningthefemaleflame.com.

Two arousal speeds exist in your bedroom, yours and your partner's. Most of the time you both want to end up highly turned on. In my practice 90% of the time it is the woman's arousal that is lagging behind the man's. He gets aroused faster and he and she are trying to get her to catch up. If you want to be aroused more fully, keep your focus on your own body and your physical feelings of pleasure. If your partner needs

It is surprising how quickly your arousal will increase when your attention is on the sensations you are feeling and not on the circling thoughts in your head.

more arousal, you can do actions that increase his or her arousal, and even when doing those actions, keep your attention registering your own body's sensations of pleasure.

BE OPEN TO THE *NEW*

One way to arouse your mind and emotions is to remain open to new experiences and ways of thinking. Getting out of an everyday mindset is marvelous. Remember Rita and Bill? They had been married for ten years and Rita enjoyed their relationship connection, yet she was not enjoying sex. Once Rita opened herself to a new experience, the positive change in their sex life happened fast. "I'd describe it like flipping a switch. It was really overnight—literally, it was overnight."

Rita said that their major turning point happened in a class they took about the energetics of relationship. A good friend had told her it was a course that was all about deepening the connection between partners. Rita and her husband had signed up for the $79 telecourse, which took place over four Tuesday evenings. The turning point occurred during the second class when they were instructed to do an exercise that asked them to imagine that each of them had two canisters of "gender essences" off to the left side of their body—

one held the "female gender essence" and the other contained the "male gender essence." They each experimented with moving one of the canisters into their body center, feeling what it was like to fully engage their male essence and then their female essence. When her husband, Bill, engaged his male essence, Rita said, she felt a charge of sexual energy between Bill and herself that was stronger than any she had felt before. "It really got my attention. I can describe it as a spark that started in my eyes, and moved down in my body, leaving me with this strong feeling of desire for Bill. It made me want to move forward and closer to him."

The very next time they made love, it was different. She "stayed open," and did not drift to her habitual thought patterns. She made a conscious decision to think differently and not think the things she had thought before. She said to herself, "Okay, here is what I always do, and I don't need to do that right now. Each time I would feel that thought come in, I would stop it."

She began to notice what was working when they made love versus what was not working. She noticed what was pleasing to her, and she realized that there was a lot more there than she had thought.

"And something shifted in Bill," she adds, "I felt like I had a different lover than I did before we started the classes. All of a sudden, it was like he understood how to touch me." When I asked her to say more, she responded that she thought it may have been their openness to the new experience of using two bodies, their physical body and their energy body when having sex—something they had learned about during the class. Perhaps that is why Bill's touch felt so much better. It may be because he was now using energy fingers, along with his physical fingers, a new concept that they were both experimenting with.

She's not sure what changed in Bill's touch, but the quality of their sex is now incredible. After orgasm they lie beside each other feeling themselves merging. She says she enjoys this blending and merging afterwards, and the energy moving in them, as much as the sex itself.

"Bill has really changed, and I'm sure that I have too. I want him so much and so strongly. We began doing all kinds of things sexually we never did before.

I did not think it was within the realm of possibility to have that fall into place with the incredible deep love and respect we have for each other. I feel like the luckiest girl in the world, certainly in my neighborhood. I feel so blessed, and wow! Who knew this was possible?"

For a few months after this change, they made love once or twice a day. This tapered off to multiple times a week—way more often than once a month, which was typical before this change.

"We lie there after we have both had orgasms, with him still inside me, and just feel the energy moving through us. It gets stronger all the time... it is this incredible melting and merging. I just can't get close enough to him. I told him the other day after we made love that I wanted him so much, that 'I just want to bite your head off like a praying mantis and have you inside of me'." She had never felt longing anywhere near that compelling before with Bill, or with anyone else.

"A lot of it for me is feeling like Bill is understanding how to touch me. It is as if he is learning that language, which is the language I know from my experience as a body worker. I had not been able to share it with him before. I don't feel like I have to be hypervigilant. I know I am going to be touched in a way that I want, so going in I am able to be more relaxed and more open, just trusting that it is going to be an enjoyable experience."

BE WILLING TO LET GO OF INHIBITIONS

Orgasms involve going over an edge. There is a moment when you lose control and you yield to the pleasure. You may make noises that don't sound like the usual you. You may moan or pant, maybe grunt or scream. Your hips may move in an aggressive or different way. You may feel yourself melting into space, or you may find yourself crying. All that is OK to do. You are safe to do this.

If you worry about how this will be perceived, remind yourself that you are in bed with someone with whom you can be fully expressive and alive. If you're in a loving, committed relationship, you probably are in bed with the person you feel the safest with in the whole world. This someone has been there many times when you have been in need. This partner has proved over time a genuine regard for you. You can reveal yourself to this person. On top of that it is quite arousing for your partner to see you sexually excited. Your partner's added excitement may arouse you even more, as well. In ongoing relationships women report feeling less inhibited as the years go by, so time, for once, is on your side.[16]

THINK SEX FRIENDLY THOUGHTS

Bring sex into your thoughts multiple times during the day. Think about sex in the morning and think about it in the afternoon. Reflect on past sexual encounters, what was the best feeling you have ever had? Remember the last time you made love and try to pinpoint your favorite part. Put your thoughts to work for you, let your thoughts rally for your sex life to be great. To fan your flame further, send a text, voice mail, or email to your partner sharing these thoughts.

16. D. Frederick et al., "What Keeps Passion Alive? Sexual Satisfaction is Associated with Sexual Communication, Mood Setting, Sexual Variety, Oral Sex, Orgasm, and Sex Frequency in a National US Study," Journal of Sex Research (2016): 1-16, doi: 10.1080/002 24499.2015.1137854.

If you are having trouble finding anything you like sexually, don't panic. Hold on. I'm going to say more about how to find what you like in the next chapter, "Optimize Your Body's Responses."

Remember That "Good" Women Do Like Sex

Good girls do like sex. If you figure out what touch makes your skin tingle or what vaginal area is most sensitive to pressure, you will not become a self-centered person. When you find the answer to the "What do I like?" question and you start to feel sexually satisfied, you will not stop thinking about other people's needs. That won't happen. You can be a responsible woman and have enthusiasm for sex. In fact, having a great sex life can make you a better person.

In the interviews I've done with women who experience enjoyable sex lives, they all reported that as they became more enthusiastic about sex, all of their relationships improved, and they became more generous and loving, not less. They appreciate and accept themselves more, and they extend that acceptance to others.

Check Out How You View Your Partner

If you are pissed off at or resentful of your partner to the extent that you no longer feel a high regard or respect for them, listen up! It's time to get outside support. Without a fundamental regard for your partner, your efforts toward a better sex life will fail.

Even though Pam resented that her husband enjoyed sex more than she did, her regard for him was intact. She knew that her husband was still a good guy. She liked him. She understood that her resentment was hers, and it did not cloud her basic assessment of him. She was able to disclose her resentment and work it out with Luis without professional help. That may not be your situation. If you have strong negative feelings toward your partner or feel paralyzed in taking action, getting a personal counselor can help.

Underneath long-held anger, resentment, and frustration there can be strong feelings of attraction. A personal counselor can help you move to a place that helps you see more options for yourself, and probably for your relationship.

Even if you cringe at the thought of a marriage/relationship counselor for financial reasons, I encourage you to make an investment of at least six sessions and then evaluate its value.

A skilled therapist can help facilitate real listening and help couples resolve seemingly impossible situations. I have seen couples discover new options when a husband finally hears how much suffering his wife has experienced with his lack of attention or appreciation. The same can occur when she understands how cruel he perceives it to be when she withholds sex or unleashes her criticism. Investing some of your time and dollars in counseling can yield many treasures, including an improved sex life.

CHAPTER NINE

Optimize Your Body's Responses

CELEBRATE YOUR BODY AND HOW IT IS GEARED FOR PLEASURE

The busyness of life sets us up to see our bodies as tools to be used, to be efficient, to accomplish tasks, to pick up the dry cleaning, to fold the laundry, to get messages off the phone and to fry the eggs. There are not many built-in messages to remind you that your body is not just a task-completer; it is your place of sensual wonder. Your body is a playground of delight, and of possible ecstasy.

Your body already has the equipment needed for exquisite sexual sensations. You may not be fully aware just how anatomically well equipped for pleasure you are, but the physical groundwork for your pleasure is built in. In this way your body is marvelous, truly marvelous. This chapter makes sure you know how well your body is equipped for sexual pleasure and includes some tips to optimize that possibility.

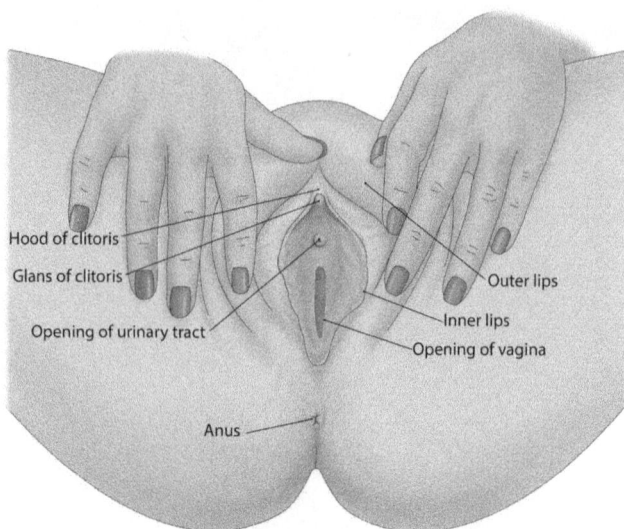

Illustration 1. Front view of Female Genitalia

On the outside of your vulva lies the glans of the clitoris: the external bump of tissue above the vagina. If you can't see it, it may be covered by a small fold of tissue. Pull that hood back and look. The clitoris has the most nerve endings of any place on your body. It is analogous to the glans of the penis (the head), which is the penis's most sensitive part with the highest concentration of nerve endings. If you did an ultrasound of your clitoris it would look surprisingly like a penis does on ultrasound.

Both these glans are sensitive to touch, sometimes extremely so. Like the penis, the clitoris has a shaft and two internal "legs," which extend down into your body along both sides of the urethra. The shaft and the legs are what cause both the penis and the clitoris to swell during arousal. They become erect. The legs of the clitoris are seven to eight times longer than the part of the clitoris you can see on the outside; each leg is somewhere around three and a half inches long.

A stand out difference between the penis and clitoris is that as far as we know, the only function of your clitoris and its 8,000

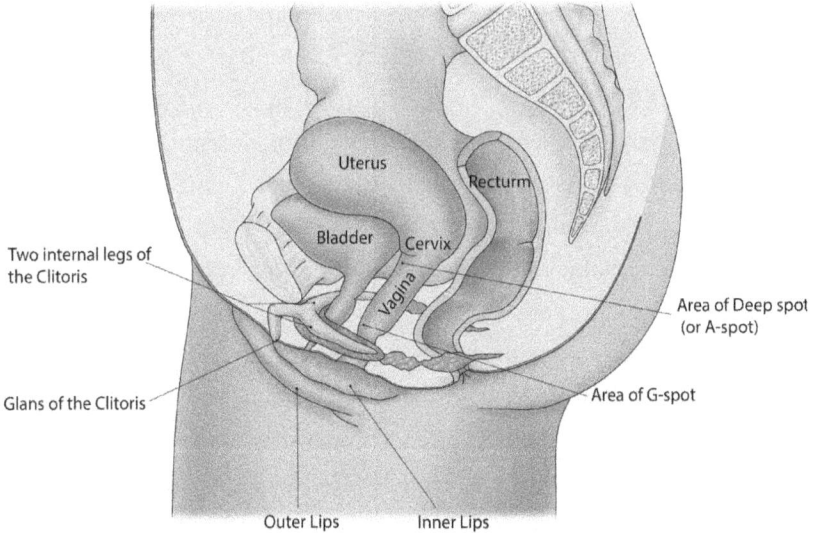

Illustration 2. Side View of Female Genitalia

nerve endings is for you to experience pleasure, sexual pleasure. Your clitoris does not secrete substances or hormones, it does not have a direct role in reproduction or urination, nor does it support any other process in your body. It is solely there for your pleasure.

Not only does your clitoris swell when you're turned on, the bulbs around the clitoris and the vascular tissue around the urethra swell too. If you look at your labia when you are aroused, you'll see they change color, often to a darker rose or a purple due to the added blood flow.

The vascular tissue surrounding the urethra is called the urethral sponge. When that is swollen, it can protrude through your upper vaginal wall, and when stimulated with a dildo, a penis, or finger, it is highly arousing. This is the G-spot area. The swelling of that sponge stimulates the legs of the clitoris, the parts you don't see, and can lead to an internal orgasm.

Deeper inside, close to the cervix is another internal area that women find exquisitely orgasmic and it is casually referred to as the

Deep spot or A-spot. This is in the upper wall of the vagina, just in front of the cervix. You don't usually feel a bump or protrusion there because it is smooth. When you are turned on it becomes a sensitive area, and pressure there, like the pressure of thrusting or a finger moving across the area, feels particularly good.

I see many women who are disappointed by not feeling a lot of sensation internally, and frustrated from not having an orgasm from intercourse alone. There is a point to make about your anatomy that can help you relax about this fact. It may shift your expectations as you explore your internal hot spots. Orgasms that include direct touch to your external clitoris are much more common than orgasms that are primarily triggered from inside the vagina. Your external clitoris is different than your other areas of sexual sensation. When you are touched there, you are making direct contact on nerve tissue. Nerves are highly sensitive, and there are more nerves there than anywhere on your body. Your response is often immediate. Touch on the G-spot and the A-spot, the hot spots inside your vagina, are not directly on nerve tissue. You won't feel things immediately there unless you had some level of arousal before you began the touch.

Also, the clitoris glans is easy to find, it is on the outside of your body and you can see it. You can't see your G-spot or Deep spot.

If you are new to exploring your internal hot spots, do it after you have some level of excitement in your body, when you are already turned on. As you explore don't expect it to feel the same as touch on the outside. It doesn't. Explore (with dildo, penis, or finger) when you have time, are open and curious, and when there is no pressure on you for a result. In general, the more aroused you are, the more blood flow in your genitals, and subsequently the more pleasure you will feel.

Make no mistake — your body is equipped for pleasure.

In addition to your awesome genitalia, your body has many other erogenous zones such as your lips, your breasts, and

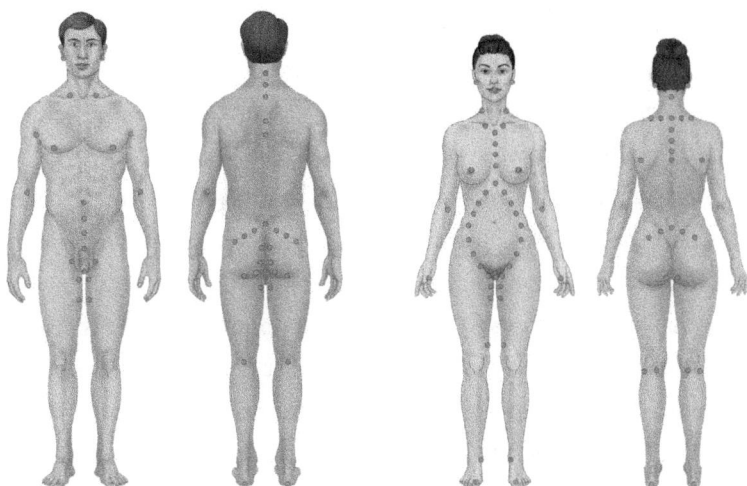

Illustration 3. Areas of Heightened Sensation

your nipples where extra nerves and blood supply and release of neurotransmitters can be highly erotic. And don't forget the largest organ in your body, your skin—the skin at the nape of your neck or your inner thigh are territories of heightened sensual delight to be explored. To give and receive sexual touch can be wonderfully erotic. Your skin is packed with multiple kinds of nerve endings that will respond to many levels of pressure and timing.

Make no mistake—you have a body designed for pleasure!

KNOW WHAT TURNS YOU ON

When women get in bed with their mates and start the touch that leads to sex, they are often starting at a zero level of arousal—possibly a one or two out of ten. The arousal level that they would find exciting enough to lead to orgasm would be a nine or a ten. That is a big jump, and it is a jump you want to know how to make.

Not many people know how to make that jump from zero to ten. A 33-year-old woman came to one of my *In the Bedroom* classes. She introduced herself saying that she was there to find out if she could have sex that was something in-between the sex she was currently having with her husband, and the sex in the popular erotic novel, *Fifty Shades of Grey.* Peals of laughter emerged from all corners of the room. The women in the class could relate.

The remarkable thing about the sex in *Fifty Shades of Grey,* in my view, was not its S & M component, it was that the book displayed the benefit of having sex with someone who knows how to increase a woman's sexual arousal. This is the standout element in the series. The sex in *Fifty Shades of Grey* did not just happen. It was sex with someone who had spent hours paying attention to what is sexually arousing to another person. Christian Grey had invested time, attention, and thousands of dollars on his sexual education. Hours were spent practicing and experimenting how to move a woman from a zero to a ten. He learned to identify increases in heart rate, to figure out which pressure of touch got his partner to breathe faster, which moans indicated she was near her edge.

DON'T THINK YOU SHOULD ALREADY KNOW

If the arousal level in your sex life does not match *Fifty Shades of Grey,* don't be down on yourself or your partner. Don't think you should already know. If you're like most of the people who come to see me, neither you nor your partner has had a single class in sexual arousal. You have not had the hours of one-on-one mentoring with uninterrupted focus and no expense spared that the fictitious Christian Grey had.

Most women I see piece together their education in sexual arousal with the bits and pieces they have stumbled upon from direct experience, or as interpreted through girlfriends, the movies, TV, *Cosmopolitan* magazine, and maybe a sister. They hope their partner has had a better education, but that is not likely. As interested as men are in getting their women excited and pleasing them, and they *are* interested in doing that, few are well informed about *how* to do it.

To fan the flame of your desire you want to identify which sexual activities work for you and then do those things.

Your partner, most likely, has had little useful education about sexual pleasure. High school sex education classes cover anatomy and physiology, pregnancy, and sexually transmitted diseases. These classes focus on real problems and risks involved with sexual activity, but they do not educate at all about how to create a peak of ecstasy. His information about your pleasure, most likely, is collected from bits too, his friends, TV, pornography, or other things he has read on the Internet, as well as what he has found to work in the past.

FINDING WHAT IS AROUSING TO YOU IS A DISCOVERY PROCESS

Finding out what is arousing to you is a process of discovery. Most of the women I talk to who have low levels of arousal have not spent time exploring their own pleasure. They have not sought to discover what works for them. Or, in some cases, they used to know, but their bodies have changed, and they need to re-explore. To fan the flame of your desire, you want to identify which activities work for you, and do them with your partner. Your arousal is a very good thing, and it is worth investing your attention to figure it out. The more you are aroused, the more excitement you will feel, and the more desire you will have.

The first thing to know is no two women are alike. You have your own personal arousal triggers. Ideas you see in the movies or

You don't decide or choose what gets you aroused or excited, you notice what actually works to turn you on.

hear from a girlfriend may not work for you. Perhaps a light touch to the side of your ribs is deliciously arousing to you. Or maybe you prefer being lifted strongly into the bed by your partner and aggressively mounted. Or a tender, personal, erotic dialogue in your ear during intercourse may be what works to get you highly aroused.

You don't get to decide or choose what gets you aroused or excited, you have to notice what works. Be yourself, relax your mind, and feel your reactions. What makes you tingly or hot? What makes you wet? Is it roses? It is his sexual advances? Is it when he does something on the edge? What gets *you* sexually excited?

Maybe romance arouses you. If so, don't judge it; work with it. Read romance novels. Watch movies with swashbuckling heroes or heroines who are swept away by love. Ask your partner to up his romantic moves. Ask to be surprised with flowers, or to have your bed littered with rose petals and an enormous number of candles lit around the room, or dine first by candlelight as a prelude.

Perhaps you'd like to role-play with him. He gets to be the Texas ranger, and you are the irresistible damsel in distress, or vice versa. As you experiment you may be surprised what excites you. Make note of it. You may not choose to do everything that excites you, but you will want to do some of them.

Watch erotic movies or read erotic literature. There is a whole genre of material out there that is specifically designed to turn you on.

Try a variety of touches and pressures, different positions, unique places, and see how you respond. Uncover what gets results, what feels good. Explore your body by yourself, and explore it together with your partner.

FEELING AROUSED WHEN YOU ARE OUT AND ABOUT

A 33-year-old client married to a musician got hot when her husband confidently described how he prepared a music student to compete in an international music contest. Another client, 44 years old, feels sexual rushes for her introverted husband when she sees him laughing and chatting with friends at a social gathering. A fifty-four-year-old woman thinks sexual thoughts when her husband, with a bare chest wearing blue jeans, sits and plays the piano for her.

What turns you on outside the bedroom? Is it when your mate does all the little things? Makes the dinner, lights the candles, or draws the bath? Volunteers to put the kids to bed? Or when he has a tool belt strapped on his waist for a building project?

FEELING AROUSED IN PRIVATE

Do you like a slow start, dancing together before you undress each other? Or is your partner's urgent hunger for you most arousing? Maybe you have noticed that slow moves and long strokes with few words make you feel more passionate. Maybe humor relaxes you enough to find your arousal. Maybe sensation is better for you with pressure on the side of the clitoris, rather than directly on top, which may feel like too much. The best way to figure these things out is to experiment.

EXPERIMENTATION IS REVEALING

Trisha was against oral sex for years until she tried it. She was surprised that she found it so pleasurable and arousing. Pam was thinking for years that orgasm should come from intercourse alone, but as she kept trying intercourse, she had no success. She thought sex was not working the way it was supposed to work and wondered what was wrong with her. When she and her husband finally experimented with direct touch to the clitoris, she had no trouble reaching orgasm. If they had not experimented, they would never have known.

GET YOUR WHOLE BODY INVOLVED

You have gates that arousal triggers have to get past to start your arousal cascade going. One good feeling leads to another good feeling, and the sensations build to orgasm. Stimulating multiple sensory channels on you at the same time can accelerate this cascade. Ask your partner to touch your nipples during intercourse, and whisper how sexy you are in your ear at the same time he is thrusting. Or ask your partner not to restrain his/her moans of enjoyment if hearing those sounds turns you on.

Women often respond to the auditory sense. Men can be more visual and may not think to offer you the words they are thinking, so ask for them. He can tell you how beautiful you look while you are moving together. At the same time you can play an erotic music track of your choice in the background. There can be sensual aromas like jasmine or patchouli in the room. Visually, you can have lots of candles flickering, and you can take in how your body parts look as they move. You want to be overwhelmed with good sensations.

When you are involved in a sexual activity and your arousal is there but not increasing, add a second and a third thing simultaneously, it can jump-start you. You are a guitar with many strings, a piano with many keys, and there may be multiple places to touch you before you find your most exquisite sound.

CONSIDER A VIBRATOR

To increase arousal, you might enjoy using a vibrator. You might especially like this if you aren't easily aroused, or if you've never had an orgasm. If you do use a vibrator, most likely your arousal will happen faster and the time to orgasm will be shorter than if you are stimulated with fingers, penis, or dildo. This is true whether you are masturbating or having sex with your partner.

Having said that, sex is so personal that using a device may not be the direction you want to take. You may not want to shorten anything in your lovemaking. Using a device may seem too mechanical or the idea of it might not turn you on at all.

Fifty-two percent of women in the US use a vibrator[17] - a marked increase from a decade ago. In my practice I find vibrators are most useful in situations where a woman feels like giving up on sex out of frustration. Her orgasms are too much work and take too long to achieve. She would rather skip sex entirely than be so frustrated. It is annoying for her to feel so unsuccessful. Avoiding sex doesn't work for her in the long run, as she misses the closeness with her partner. Her partner is frustrated too. When she uses a vibrator and orgasms, she feels less frustrated. She and her partner become closer, and she starts to enjoy sex again.

Deborah started to have a sexual "problem" at age 63, after she was diagnosed with breast cancer. Right after the diagnosis, Deborah did not have sex. She turned inward and for months she focused her attention on healing herself. The chemo and radiation took six months, and another six months passed before she thought much about sex at all. Then she realized she missed it. She missed the closeness with her husband, Mike, and the sex act itself. She

---

17. D. Herbenick et al., "Prevalence and Characteristics of Vibrator Use by Women in the United States: Results from a Nationally Representative Study," The Journal of Sexual Medicine 7, no. 6 (2009): 1857-1866.

missed the penetration and the response it brought about in her.

When she and Mike had intercourse again, it hurt. Her vaginal tissues felt dry and thin. Her vaginal walls felt like they had shrunk. The longer the penetration went on and the more thrusting there was, the more it hurt, both during intercourse and after.

Deborah spoke to her oncologist about the pain and the dryness, and she recommended some remedies to deal with the dryness—an Estring (a circular tube placed in the vagina near the cervix that releases 7.5 mg of estrogen daily into the vagina) and a lubricant.

Deborah used the Estring for three months. She found a massage oil that she liked to help her lubricate well enough to keep the pain away. However, if sex took too long to complete, she was still in pain.

The whole of you wants to be captivated during sex, so find out what captures the whole of you.

One day she had lunch with a friend she had not seen in years. As they were catching up, the friend revealed that she had designed a couple's vibrator and brought it to market, a couple's vibrator "designed to make women orgasm more quickly." Deborah's ears perked up. Orgasm more quickly—she wanted to orgasm more quickly. She asked her friend for the details.

The FixSation™ device is a thin, smooth couples vibrator. It is designed to fill in the gap between the man and woman's pelvises, and is held in place externally, above the clitoris, by lacy lingerie straps. When thrusting occurs with the male on top, the device applies vibration and pressure to the external clitoris. Today there are multiple types of couple's vibrators on the market.

Deborah got the device, and she and Mike experimented with it. Using it allows her to orgasm quickly, within five minutes of intercourse. Her husband climaxes then too. They are back to their mutually-satisfying lovemaking, without prolonged wear and tear on her thin vaginal tissue. She is experiencing the penetrative sex act she enjoys, having the orgasms she enjoys, with no pain during or after. This shorter time to orgasm worked for her.

WHAT TO DO IF YOU DON'T KNOW WHAT TURNS YOU ON

If asking the question, "What turns me on?" draws a blank, you are not alone. Many women tell me that their partner asks what they like, and they don't know what to say. They are stumped. They were hoping he or she would figure it out for them. But the truth is, this is an essential question for you. What pleases *you* really matters to your sex life.

If you can't think of a thing you like about sex, start first by identifying non-sexual things you enjoy—walking barefoot in warm sand, lemon meringue pie, the color teal, or the smell of coffee. Enjoying anything is a response from your being that shows your attraction toward it. It is a whole person response. It is not merely a thought. The whole of you wants to be captivated during sex, so you want to find out what captures the whole of you.

The part of you that registers what you like works like a muscle, it gets stronger the more you use it. To have great sex, you want to develop your *pleasure* muscle. To do this notice when you are captivated by the way you feel, when you are pleased, or tickled. Notice what brought you to this state of feeling absolutely delighted.

In the bedroom the action is about you and what you like. It is about your pleasure.

After you have found some general likes, go on from there and notice what gets you sexually excited. No judgment, just notice. Write down what you notice. Push yourself to be as specific as possible. Remember what has pleased you in the past, even decades ago, and see if it still works. This is part of your arousal map. Your arousal map is made up of the things that get you sexually excited and you want to know what those things are.

If you cannot identify anything that arouses you, keep the question alive inside. As time goes on, you might begin to notice the triggers that get you thinking juicy thoughts. Even if it is just a flash of a sexual thought, make a note of it.

Many of the women I work with spend their days feeling responsible for other people—their staff, children, company, ageing parents. The schedule for their day is not set up to register what they like, but rather to track the tasks that they need to accomplish for others. Some women are so accustomed to meeting others' needs that the things they like, even small things, don't figure into their day. Their pleasure muscle is rarely flexed. Start flexing yours. Put things in your day just for you. Think about what you want and make it happen. For example, if you like sunshine on your face, figure out where you can take your morning break and step out into the sun. If you love to have your feet massaged, set up an appointment with a massage therapist, or ask your partner or a friend.

In the bedroom, the action is about you and what you like. It is not about anyone else's pleasure. Flexing that pleasure muscle in small, daily ways will add to your ability to find what turns you on in the bedroom.

Exercise - A Libido Accelerant

If you want an effective and inexpensive libido charger, try aerobic exercise. Aerobic exercise increases the sexual arousal you experience. It activates your sympathetic nervous system, which increases the arousal of your genitals and supports you having a good time. The effect can be immediate, as aerobic exercise twenty or thirty minutes before an erotic activity has been shown to increase vaginal blood flow in women with low desire.[18]

Besides this direct physical increase in blood flow to the genitals, women who exercise three or four times a week tell me they like their bodies more than when they don't exercise. They feel sexier and more vibrant. Women who do regular movement practices, such as dance, running, Tai chi, Pilates, or yoga feel more present and aware of physical sensations in their body. Exercise, as you likely know, promotes your overall health in multiple other ways—reduces stress, increases metabolism, relieves depression, increases self-esteem, protects heart and lungs, and decreases your risk of cancer, diabetes and other conditions. The list goes on. Exercise works. To add to the probability of you having a great sex life, find an exercise activity that you enjoy—one that makes you feel good, not just afterwards, but while you're doing it. It could be dancing the tango, or doing Zumba or Nia, or taking a walk in a park or around a lake. Maybe you'd enjoy working out on an elliptical *Aerobic exercise* or rowing machine while you watch romantic *is an inexpensive* movies. Find an exercise that personally pleases *libido accelerant.* you and then enjoy moving that wonderful body of yours.

OVER-THE-COUNTER APHRODISIACS WITH POSSIBILITY

B vitamins: If you feel low in mood, energy, stamina, and libido, you may benefit from taking a B complex to help your brain make those friendly neurotransmitters, like dopamine and serotonin. Also, your body uses B6 to make libido enhancing estrogen and testosterone, so pick a B complex that has 50 to 100 mg of B6 in it, not only 2 mg.

---

18. C. M. Meston and B.B. Gorzalka, "Differential Effects of Sympathetic Activation on Sexual Arousal in Sexually Dysfunctional and Functional Women," Journal of Abnormal Psychology 105 (1996): 582-591.

Note: Around twenty percent of the women I see experience nausea while taking B vitamins, especially when consumed on an empty stomach, so take it after breakfast. A few women will discover they have too much energy while taking B vitamins. If you feel this way reduce to a 50 mg capsule instead of 100 mg.

Other vitamins and minerals like vitamin E, zinc, and magnesium are known to be essential for normal sexual function. We lack any data that says supplementing with them will increase a woman's desire, and yet we know they are vital.

In 2015, a review of the available research on natural aphrodisiacs was published.[19] This review was done to find out if there was any evidence to support all the claims of sexual wonder. Turns out that Fenugreek, Korean Red Ginseng, Maca, L-arginine and Tribulus Terrestris are plant products that did show supporting evidence, even if the evidence was limited in scope. I have included a few details from this review of research below.

I include this section because of all the women I see who want a "natural" treatment for their sex life. There are many of you who don't want a drug, but do experiment with over-the-counter herbs. Because we don't have enough evidence-based data to generate guidelines for safe use you are left somewhat on your own. I say somewhat as there are naturopaths, herbalists, and nutritionists who are well educated in the potential of these plant products. These over-the-counter products are available to everyone, and yet they are not safe for everyone to use. The comments below outline for you what is known about these products from medical research.

Fenugreek: Fenugreek is an herb, often used in Ayurvedic medicine, which contains building blocks used to create estrogen and testosterone. A 2015 study showed that Fenugreek improved the arousal, lubrication, and satisfaction in premenopausal women.

---

19. E. West and M. Krychman, "Natural Aphrodisiacs – A Review of Selected Sexual Enhancers," Sexual Medicine Reviews 3, no. 4 (2015): 279-288.

There were minor intestinal side effects. The dose used in the study was 300 mg twice a day. Fenugreek should not be used by people taking blood-thinning medication (anticoagulants), or by women with hormonally active cancers.

Maca: Maca is a root vegetable from Peru and has long been used for fertility in the Andean culture. Three out of four of the random clinical trials mentioned in this review did show positive effects on sexuality. Study doses ranged from 1.5 to 3 grams of Maca a day. Its mechanism of action is not fully understood. It is known to not alter estrogen and testosterone levels as Fenugreek does. It does contain phytoestrogens, plant-based compounds that can inhabit the estrogen receptors in your body. This can be a good thing or a bad thing depending on who you are, your hormonal status, whether you have cancer, the medications you are on, and many other things that researchers are currently trying to decipher. Maca is well tolerated. We do not yet have data on what doses are optimal or safe for women to take.

Ginseng: Korean Red Ginseng is an herb that has been shown in one double-blind study to heighten arousal in menopausal women. It works by encouraging the release of nitric oxide, which improves blood flow in the clitoris and vaginal walls. (This is the same biochemical pathway that is augmented by Viagra, Cialis and similar medications.) Ginseng has been shown to be estrogenic, so it should be avoided by women with hormonally active cancers, and by women who have bleeding disorders or are on anticoagulant medications.

Tribulus Terrestris: This herb contains a compound which converts to DHEA. DHEA, you remember, is a building block for your testosterone. This review found two, randomized placebo-controlled studies that demonstrated improvement in female sexual function using this herb. The herb was well-tolerated and caused minor intestinal side effects.

Horny Goat Weed (Traditional Chinese Medicine herb), Potency Wood (Brazilian herb) Damiana Leaf (extract from a Mexican shrub), and Gingko (tree used in Traditional Chinese Medicine) have promise, yet lack research. Yohimbine (parts from an African plant) is a strong aphrodisiac, yet its side effects can be life threatening, so it is not recommended for any over-the-counter use.

L-arginine, a common amino acid, is taken by many men and some women for a Viagra-like effect. It is a precursor to nitric oxide and nitric oxide causes blood vessels to dilate and fill with blood all over your body, including the clitoral and vaginal areas. There is significant evidence that L-arginine is helpful in producing firmer erections in men. Research on L-arginine by itself in women is lacking. There is a small double-blind study of 108 women that showed an increase in sexual desire and sexual satisfaction after taking the supplement ArginMax. This is a multi-ingredient supplement which has L-arginine in it, along with a variety of vitamins and herbs, some of which we have just mentioned: Korean Ginseng, Ginkgo, and Damiana Leaf.

CHAPTER TEN

Empower Your Communication

In June 2016 there was a headline in *The Wall Street Journal,* "Women May Be More Interested in Sex Than You Think." Curious, I read on. It was a discussion of research that had just been published on how difficult it is to perceive accurately whether your partner wants to have sex.[20] The study subjects were all couples in long-term heterosexual relationships. Women predicted accurately their partners' interest in sex, and men missed women's interest one third of the time. Multiple theories were put forward to account for this misperception, all interesting and intelligent. Some of the discussion was that the women's indication that she was a *yes for sex* was communicated so indirectly that it was not interpreted as a *yes* by their partner. What I want to note is the importance of sending sexual signals to your partner that he or she won't miss and also

20. A. Muise, et al., "Not in the Mood? Men Under- (Not Over-) Perceive Their Partner's Sexual Desire in Established Intimate Relationships," Journal of Personality and Social Psychology 110, no. 5 (2016): 725-742, doi:http://dx.doi.org/10.1037/pspi0000046.

won't misinterpret. This chapter, "Empower Your Communication," includes strategies on how to add clarity and power to your exchanges about sex.

Say No to Sex Clearly and with Confidence

Living with a mate who wants more sex than you do can become a high-pressure situation with no apparent right answer. You don't want to say no again; you are tired of saying no. You are tired of that defensive role, of feeling like a stingy female metering out the goodies. Yet you don't want to have sex when you're not into it. Neither choice is a good one for you.

Let's revisit the story of Sofia and Nathan. Nathan wanted sex once a day or more. Sofia did not. Sofia was trying to figure out her own level of desire, without Nathan's influence. The greatest help for Sofia in finding her sexual desire was acquiring the skill to say no to sex clearly and with confidence. Once she was able to tell Nathan no without feeling guilt or yielding to pressure, it helped her find her yes. Sofia learned that men could accept a no. She found she was able to say no and realized it did not end their relationship.

Living with a mate who wants more sex than you do can become a high-pressure situation with no apparent right answer.

"He could take it," she said. His yearning for her did not go away, and he did not go away. Sofia saying no clearly was relaxing for them both. Neither one had to wallow in the indecisiveness of a wavering, fuzzy choice. Before, she had feared that if she said no, he would think she was not interested in him, or think that she was not a sexual person. She had figured that saying no would be awkward or difficult. But in fact, Sofia says it has been the opposite. Saying no instead of skirting around the issue is way more positive for her.

Saying no, Sofia found, added to her ability to say yes. When she felt a clear yes, she could give herself over to the moment completely. She and Nathan then had sexual experiences that she treasured. Finding her yes grew when she learned to say no with confidence.

HOW TO SAY NO

Be direct and clear. No is no. And when you say no keep your sexiness alive. Just because sex is a no for you in one moment, there's no need to dial down your sexuality. You are an alive and vibrant being. It is you, a dynamic woman who is saying not now. You do not have to take on the persona of a matronly, uptight, or apologetic female because you are saying no. You can say no, not now with your eyes sparkling. You also don't need to undress in the closet hoping to avoid turning him on. If it is not the moment to be sexual, communicate that.

HOW TO SAY NO IF YOU HAVE SAID NO A LOT

One way that I have seen work to keep you closer together about sex, especially if you are the partner with lower desire, is this: when you do say no to sex, add a promise of a future yes at that same time, and mean it. For example:

I have to go work. Come shower with me now and we can play tonight.

No sex now, but looking forward to Saturday morning.

Saying no is a sensitive declaration. It can be destructive if your partner has resentment about your lack of availability for sex. Couples with different levels of desire for sex are in the opposite of a win-win situation; it is extremely painful and disempowering for both. Be respectful of your partner and their feelings of frustration or powerlessness. If resentment is pervasive get professional help in sorting this out.

Alert: Be sure if you actually make a promise to have sex, that you keep that promise. Sex is so centrally important for some men and women it is not a promise you want to break.

When Something Works to Arouse You, Don't Keep It to Yourself

Whatever it is, when something works in bed, don't keep it to yourself. With your words or your moans, let your partner know you are turned on. You can say, "More there. Yes! That's it."

When things are not working, let him know too. If his hand is slightly off the right spot, move it. If the pressure is too strong, adjust your body or his.

Don't do it as a frustrated woman, or a stern teacher, do it as a sexy female who is aroused and wanting to be more aroused. You are on the same team, working together to make sex exciting for both of you. If you don't know what touch or position you want, but you know what he or she is doing isn't working, communicate your desire to experiment, "Let's try here," or "Touch me here." Take his hand and place it where you can explore. Move it in the rhythm that feels good to you. Small communications like these build on each other.

If squeezing your nipples is more arousing than kissing them, tell him to squeeze them. If you know the kind of passion in the kiss you want, show him. Kiss him the way you want to be kissed.

Saying no, Sofia found, added to her ability to say yes. When she felt a clear yes she could give herself over to the moment completely.

Tell him in your aroused, passionate (not angry or critical) voice that this is how you love to kiss.

Don't take it personally if you have to tell him again the next time. Persist. When he sees what awakens in you when you get fully excited his memory will improve.

Be direct and positive. A man's macho self can take it. They can take your honesty. They want you to be excited, they are more open to change than you think. They don't know what to do to get you excited, so tell them.

You might think it would feel awkward to disclose the touch you like after many years of living with something that didn't really turn you on. The women in these interviews said it didn't unfold that way. The positive nature of their closeness and eroticism was so apparent to both of them, and so desired, that any feeling of awkwardness disappeared quickly.

If your partner is female, communicate with her in the language that would work for you, whether you are using the language of touch or words. Watch and listen to her responses closely.

Sometimes your partner's focus on your orgasm can feel like pressure that you don't want. Pam originally felt her husband's desire for her to have an orgasm was a demand that left her feeling that she had to hurry up and come. She did not want to do that. She told him that she was OK not coming every time; she would rather make love slowly and be into it, and not worry about an orgasm. If in the moment your orgasm is not your focus, let your partner know so you are both on the same page.

MAKE SOMETHING INTERESTING HAPPEN BECAUSE YOU HAVE THE POWER TO DO THAT

Many women have no desire for sex until after they are aroused. Once aroused, they remember how delicious sex is, and they want it—they can then want it a lot. If you experience desire after you are aroused, rather than before, you'll respond to your partner's advances, but you won't feel much of a trigger to initiate sex yourself. This puts you in an inactive stance a lot of the time. Many of the women I see aren't used to this inactive place and/or they don't care for it. How do you even get something interesting going when you feel neutral most of the time?

This progression from arousal to desire vs. having desire first and then going on to feel aroused is so frequently reported by women that sex researcher Dr. Rosemary Basson, MD, from Vancouver, BC, created a model for the sexual cycle of females that includes this possibility.[21] The previously existing model, which you may have seen in your human sexuality classes, has desire always occurring prior to arousal. This original model may match your experience of spontaneous desire; when you are the one hungry for sex and you are the one moving towards your partner with sex on your mind. The Basson Model includes the possibility that women's desire for sex can come after things heat up. This model captures the experience of the women in my office who say "I never think about sex anymore, I say yes because I know it is important to him. After we get going I remember how good it feels and then I want to keep going." This model acknowledges that many women do begin being sexual from a neutral starting place. They can go on from there to have terrifically satisfying lovemaking.

If you are in a neutral place you are not stuck there. Even if your partner is not doing all the little things to get you interested (i.e. building your responsive desire) you can still add a punctuation mark to your week. You don't have to feel a sexual urge before you take action. Don't make yourself wait for that. Remember how you feel when you get sexually excited and grab him or her by the shirttail (or make a love date). Start something interesting with your partner because you can. You have the power to do that. Celebrate that power. This pro-active stance can create a positive ripple for you both.

---

21. Diagrams of both of these models are in the Appendices at the back of the book.

CHAPTER ELEVEN

Use Your Feminine Sexuality to Spice Things Up

ACCEPT HOW ATTRACTIVE YOU ARE TO YOUR PARTNER

Not too long ago, my husband and I were sitting at the dinner table having a conversation about our favorite Hollywood actors with our younger son who was twenty-six at the time. He said his favorite actress was Penelope Cruz. "Her voice," he said with wistful longing, "I just want to be around it. I wouldn't care if she were crazy mad and yelling at me, I want to be close to that voice."

"There it is," I thought "that attractive force that women have with men."

Men want to be close to women. It is so real and so persistent. I think that women don't realize how persistent that desire is. Your man is like a moth to a flame, and you are the flame. You are the one your partner wants to be close to. You are it. It is your body and your curves, and the beauty and mystery of your feminine nature that attracts your partner. You are the flame.

HIGHLIGHT YOUR FEMALENESS

Any time, any day you have a myriad of ways to use this attractive power you have to increase sexual possibilities. One way to do this is to highlight your body. When you accent your curves, or emphasize your femaleness, you create a good kind of tension that can ignite desire in both of you. Or you can hide your curves, your breasts, and hips, and keep the tension down. You can wear a sheer, lacy nightgown that shows your silhouette, or you can wear flannel pajamas. A choice that accentuates your femininity is more likely to ignite passion in your partner.

Highlighting her femininity was central to Trisha sparking the change in her sex life. As you may recall from Part 1, Trisha had lost her libido at menopause. Her sex life had become boring, and she came to my *In the Bedroom* series for help. At the end of the first class, I showed slides with pictures of ten low- or no-cost things a woman could do to spark an immediate sexual charge with her partner.

Ten Low to No Cost Things You Can Do to Spark an Immediate Sexual Charge

Stage your bedroom for a romantic *event*.
Make a sexual promise and keep it.
Interrupt your partner with one agenda only.
Give a sensual massage.
Break the rules.
Dress for sex.
Deliver a message written in lipstick.
Flash a body part, accidentally or with emphasis.
Role play with characters you enjoy.
Send suggestive voice mails or texts – both ways.

Right after class, Trisha came up to me and asked if she could have a different assignment. "You need to understand, I don't have any libido. I can't do these things. I don't have any desire for sex," she said.

"Do them anyway," I said. I wasn't being unkind. I knew that the best way for her to find her libido was to take action.

You are it. You are the treasure. It is your body and your curves and the beauty and mystery of your feminine nature that attracts your partner.

The following week Trisha was the first to raise her hand. She reported that she had done the assignment and picked something from the list, and she was shocked. She had dressed up in a sexy way, put on lipstick and eye makeup, and gone on a date with her husband. She flirted and they had fun. She already felt juicy again.

"I was so surprised. I didn't believe I could. I did all those things thinking nothing would happen. Now I am looking forward to sex with my husband!" Three months later, I followed up with her. She referred to her sex life as "hot."

"I did not know that I could control feeling horny through my mind, through thinking about sex, and through dressing up like I used to when I was sixteen or twenty-six and feeling beautiful. I think the key for me is really attention. Like you said, I can create that same feeling of hormonal need now, after menopause, by giving my attention to sex and feeling sexy. Part of all that is getting dressed up a little bit and going out somewhere in the evening, which we know isn't the sexual part but we do it anyway. I like getting dressed up, knowing full well what's coming later, and flirting, and making an event of the whole process so that I am feeling quite juicy by the time we even hit the bedroom. All of those things have rekindled my desire. I actually feel horny again!"

Sounds kind of trivial and superficial to remember to dress sexily again. Luckily we have great bodies, so why not use them and dress sexily and not worry about the fact that I'm sixty-two years old, or believe that I should dress like sixty-two. No, I should not! To be the seductress in the bedroom, it's the whole process—the way I dress and look, to the way the bedroom is decorated, to creating events, to having dates. Maybe going out for a six course meal, maybe going out for a martini, or something, but somewhere a little elegant."

Overall, Trisha said her sex life has gone from boring to hot; in fact, her word now is "uninhibited." She gives herself over to the experience of sex. Her mind quits and she allows her body to take over. There is no control, and she can get lost in the experience. It feels like freedom and openness to her. It feels like coming home.

She gets that luscious experience of oneness, the feeling that there is no separation between her and her husband.

Our little secret of what we've done here together in the bedroom, which was a big step in our intimacy, spills over to appreciation in all the other areas of our lives as well."

"I did a lap dance for him, which was great. I got dressed up and he chose the music, he arranged soft lighting in the room so it wasn't too bright. The whole series (*In the Bedroom*) gave me permission to be erotic to do all that. It was wonderful. We went out together to get the stockings and the garter belt. He loves such things. And it's just fun. It is about bringing the fun back in."

Connecting sexually has brought in more tenderness and respect. "We are both far more loving in the little ways throughout the day. It is just sweet. It really has improved in small ways which is lovely. There's a wonderful sense of gratitude for each other. Our little secret of what we've done here together in the bedroom, which was a big step in intimacy, spills over to appreciation in all the other ways as well."

Trisha found that if she and her husband got into "work mode" for days at a time, they would schedule a date, and the good sexual tension returned. If Trisha missed sex first, she asked her husband to create a date. She liked it when he asked her to go on a date. His expression of desire for her added more romance, and she found romance arousing.

There was another physical piece that added to Trisha's pleasure. Ted's erection had been getting softer in the past few years. They went together to see his primary care physician and got a Cialis prescription. Since using it, Trisha can orgasm again from being on top during intercourse. She had enjoyed this a lot in the past, and though she had added in oral sex successfully, having more variety of sexual positions was a positive.

Engage in the Dynamic Exchange of Attention and Sex

This intentional addition of feminine energy into the mix is a recipe that works to increase desire in both the male and the female. Even in relationships that have suffered decades-long dry spells, it can turn around quickly, even immediately. It takes only one person in the couple to get things going. If you, as a woman, claim your sexuality and express it, you can get your partner's attention.

Patty and Paul Richards introduced me to this dynamic years ago in their work and subsequent book *Wild Attraction, a Ruthlessly Practical Guide to Extraordinary Relationship.* In this model of relationship, "Women want men who will provide sophisticated and positive attention, and men want women who will provide sexuality and charge."[22]

Don't think too much about this dynamic, it may sound impossible to you or too traditional, but do try it. It felt counter-intuitive for Trisha to dress up, use lipstick, and flirt when she had

---

22. Paul Richards and Patricia Richards, Wild Attraction: The Energetic Facts of Life (Ashland, Oregon: Chelsion Press, 2008), 115.

no desire for sex, but she did it. She re-engaged with her sexuality and when she did their sex life shifted.

Rita did it too. Rita (who is now the *luckiest girl in her neighborhood*) began to accent her femaleness *after* she and her husband connected sexually. She now wears boots, belts, and picks blouses with necklines that flatter her chest. She chooses more feminine clothes and displays more confidence. She now likes sex with her husband and wants to keep what they have found active in their lives. Doing these seemingly small things keeps it alive.

She recognizes that her husband Bill is visual, and he enjoys it when she dresses up.

Also, she plays games to draw his attention to her. "I do things during the day just to get his attention, little sexy moves (wiggle my hips or lift my skirt up a few inches) and he notices. We are building charge (sexual tension) and noticing each other in different ways. There is this constant element of fun and energy throughout the day. All of this is part of our answer."

The shift in her sex life changed how she dressed and how she related to the world. "I am now aware of my sexuality and aware of my capacity to enjoy it. It is like I am part of this club that I was not privy to before. Not only that, I can carry it into my work with men and know that I am attractive. I have really changed my physical appearance. I make a very conscious effort to put a lot more care and attention into how I dress."

Rita has a friend who taught her about a dressing plan where you keep adding clothing elements until your outfit reaches a ten. She goes for a ten most days.

You can do this sexuality dance if you are a woman in a relationship with a woman. What role you have, either giving attention or being the recipient of her attention, varies between the two of you. Which one of you is displaying more of their feminine nature and being receptive can change. We have female and male aspects to our natures and the amount of an aspect we display can change moment to moment. I have seen intimacy increase when one female partner claims more of their so-called masculine aspects, for example, initiation and action, and the other takes the posture of being on the receiving end of those actions.

Own That You Want His Attention and Keep the Dance Going

Research has shown in study after study that women have more sexual desire at the beginning of a relationship than as it progresses. This finding persists whether the women in the study are in their twenties or their sixties. There are many reasons for a decline in desire, and I have outlined many of them in the first two chapters. I want to point out to you that this dance of sexuality, which often starts off with strong energy, fades over time and can parallel the drop in libido many women experience as a relationship progresses. See if you relate to this description: At the beginning of dating you may have focused on what to wear, how your hair should be, which necklace to put on. Your friends may have helped you pick out your outfit for those first few dates, or suggested topics to talk about. You may have flirted and teased. You conveyed in your voice and your actions that you were an interesting and available female. You were engaged in the dynamics of possibility that passed between you and your partner, and you were invested in showing it. When you were first together your partner may have paid a lot of attention to you, and tried to figure out what would be the most interesting date he could take you on. He was fascinated by your smile and presence. He was intrigued, and may have brought you gifts or surprises.

As the months and years went on, you may have dressed with less care, flirted and teased less often. After all, you figured you already had him. You did not have to capture his attention. Not that you lost interest in him. You still think he is great, but you feel you don't have to do anything special to keep him. He forgot to notice your mood or compliment you on your dress as often. He stopped trying to figure out what he could do that was interesting to you. He was not as genuinely curious about your day. You focused well together on household projects or children, but did not give much thought to the signals that you sent back and forth between you. You didn't go on dates often, and when you did you were not dressing to interest him the way you were initially. Maybe on your birthday he started paying attention to what you liked, but the day-to-day attention was less frequent, and the intimacy and excitement you experienced dwindled.

WHAT TO DO IF YOUR RELATIONSHIP IS TOO GOOD TO LEAVE, AND YET IS NOT EXCITING

If your relationship is not exciting to you now, take a look at this dynamic and see if it is playing out in your relationship. I would underline this ten times: *When a man (or the partner choosing to express more 'maleness') frees up his/her attention and places it in a positive and attentive way on his wife or partner, and when a woman confidently claims and expresses her sexuality, things in the bedroom heat up.*

As simple as it sounds, doing these things is not intuitive. Ask yourself, is your partner paying attention to you in a way that is positive and nourishing? Do you feel included in his/her attention most of the time even when you don't need anything? If he or she has stopped, what can you do to get that dynamic going again? Your part of the action has been the focus of this book. There is another half of the dance that involves how the man can start things up with you; how he can get things going, or keep things going, even when you are not feeling engaged sexually. The nice thing that I have observed is this: though it takes two to tango, it only takes one person to start things rolling in that direction. You can be that one. Own your femininity confidently, and make it more real and visible to yourself and to your partner. It is not just your body you are sharing, it is your aesthetic, your motion, your being.

CHAPTER TWELVE

Set the Stage for Delicious Sexual Events

Make the bedroom a place that turns you on – a room that reminds you to feel your sensuality as soon as you walk into it. Declare this room to be only about the sensual wonder and magic that is possible between your partner and you. Even if you're not feeling that magic in the relationship yet, make the room feel and appear as if you are.

CREATE THE ENVIRONMENT THAT INVITES THE SEXUAL YOU TO SHOW UP

Imagine a room decorated to match the sex life that you want to have. You can create this by the use of textures, colors, lighting, and accessories. Start by selecting a theme that makes you feel tender, open, and excited. If exotic places create interest for you, include elements of exotic décor. If a romantic style is what revs you up, create that. If clean lines and simple surroundings make you feel most open for love, then keep the room décor understated.

A quick Google search of exotic, romantic, or contemporary bedrooms will yield endless decorating ideas that you can use to ignite your style of romance. I am not an interior decorator, so I either use pictures of what others have created or ask my décor savvy friends to come over and help me. You may want to ask your friends too. After you explore and recognize which theme works for you, put your plan into action.

The décor should draw your eye to the bed and should elicit the idea of sex or sleep. Nothing else. The bedroom is not a home office, a laundry-sorting station, or a TV room.

Even if the kids still sleep in your room at times, your kids' stuff, including family pictures, should be placed elsewhere. This is an adult space. It's your play area. The bedroom needs to reflect an intimate, safe place where you can temporarily step out of the "mom" mindset. The other rooms in the house can be family rooms.

Get rid of everything that is not linked with either intimacy or rest. *Be ruthless!*

Textures: Use fabrics that invite you to want to touch them. Create a "want to stay a while" atmosphere by adding layers of silk, faux furs, mohair, cashmere, fine linens, and other soft, velvety cottons. Make it a sensual playground.

Colors: The colors of the sheets, bedspreads, walls, and pillows should compliment your eyes, hair, and skin. You are the beauty in the room. Showcase yourself at your sensuous best!

If you don't know what your best colors are, you can hire a color expert who can advise you or go to the bookstore and find a good book like the one referenced below.[23]

Lighting: Most women agree that bright light will dampen a sultry mood faster than things disappear when you hit delete on the

---

23. Carla Mason Mathis and Helen Villa Connor, The Triumph of Individual Style: A Guide to Dressing Your Body, Your Beauty, Your Self (New York: Fairchild Publications, 2002), 112-153.

keyboard. Replace harsh white light bulbs with soft pink ones. If you can, add a dimmer switch. Use candles too. The flickering of candlelight can add to the feel of romance in the room and provide a gorgeous forgiving glow to your skin. If you're worried about burning down the house, there are many electronic candles on the market that can mimic the same effect. If you

Own your femininity with confidence, and make it more real and visible to yourself and to your partner. It is not just your body you are sharing; it is your aesthetic, your motion, your being

want to really shake things up, occasionally introduce strobe lights and/or black lights to the mix.

Accessorize: Add framed, romantic, or sensual pictures of the two of you together to remind you of what this room is about. Add accents of curved vases, sculptures, or other shapes that suggests a sensuous body.

If you like music, collect songs or albums on your iPod or CD player that make you feel sexy. If you have yet to compile a collection of songs that get you in the mood, start listening to music with this question in mind, "What songs make me feel sensually alive and excited?" Create a way in which you can quickly access and play those songs when the mood strikes.

Couples that take the time to set the mood through lighting a candle and playing music have been shown to be the couples that have more passion and satisfaction in their sexual relationships over time.

Make sure to delight all of your senses. Sensual smells can be provocative, and using scented candles or essential oil diffusers can add to your relaxation and arousal. Essential oils that are used to increase arousal include jasmine, cinnamon, ginger, rose, vanilla, patchouli, and ylang-ylang. You probably won't like all of them, so try several to see which ones turn you on.

If you use oils, lubricants, contraceptives, or other devices, find an easy-access and aesthetic way to store them. Also, include benches, stools, and cushions in the furnishings. They can facilitate different activities and positions. You also may place mirrors in strategic places for visual stimulation.

You don't have to spend a lot of money. You can find many of these items at popular discount stores.

You'll know your room is ready when you can answer these three questions with an emphatic "Yes!"

- Is your bedroom a place that looks like it is ready for a romantic and sexual encounter?
- Does it inspire you to feel sensually activated?
- Does the décor accent your beauty, your skin tone, eye color, and hair color?

Claiming your bedroom as a special place to enjoy your sex life is a concrete way to declare that your sex life has your attention, and that it is important. Committing to this one change, creating an inviting sensual bedroom space creates a ripple effect that can be bigger than expected.

If your lovemaking space delights your senses, you are much more likely to show up in it with all your senses ready to be delighted. Remember, surrounding yourself with what's arousing and interesting to you is central to having a great sex life.

CHAPTER THIRTEEN

Go Fan That Flame!

IT IS TIME TO EMBARK ON THE JOURNEY

The ingredients for a great sex life may already be right in front of you. You don't need a new partner or a different body. You need to connect the dots with what you already have. It is all about taking action. The women in the success stories made the risky move and the decisions they needed so that they could have a better experience. They experimented and found out what aroused them. It was not always comfortable, but the actions were absolutely doable. Their desire for change percolated through their lives differently, but each woman took action. When she heard about a class, she took it. When she heard about a device, she tried it. When she had dryness, she spoke to her physician. When her husband had an affair, she faced her part in their disconnect. These women who had been waiting for change, sometimes for decades, became action takers.

In the end, these women did not wait for life to give them

great sex; they took action to get it, and a whole new world opened up for them. The adjectives that described their feelings about sex changed from bored, disinterested, uptight, reserved, avoidant, in pain, confused, and resentful to enthusiastic, positive, experimental, excited, transformed, hot, and lucky. They didn't need to change partners to do it.

In spite of all the research that says women's interest fades over time, it is not inevitable. In 2016 research was published that re-evaluated data collected online with 38,747 participants in long-term relationships, 15,886 of the participants were women. The study looked at what keeps passion alive over time.[24] Thirty-eight percent of the women in the study said their passion was as high as when their relationship began. Thirty-two percent of the men said the same thing. Turns out these couples that were equally as passionate now as when they first met did a number of things that the couples that had lost their passion did not do, or did not do as much. Couples with passion had more variety in what they did sexually, they communicated more about sex, and they did more mood setting (e.g., candles, dimmed light, music, sexy talk). These actions made their passion last over time.

Now is the time for you to take action. What are you going to do? Which of the five areas do you wish to try first?

- Arouse your mind and emotions.
- Optimize your body's responses.
- Empower your communication.
- Use your femininity to spice things up.
- Set the stage for the most delicious sexual encounters.

You choose where you start. Most likely one area will seem more compelling than the others. Maybe start there. Or if you want to start with one that is less personal and has some shopping fun, start

---

24. D. Frederick, "What Keeps Passion," 1-16.

with creating a bedroom that works for you. If you are stalled by feelings of resentment, your first action may be to get a counselor, or perhaps your first will be to make a medical appointment to rule out the physical things I outlined in Part 2. Regardless what it is, or even if it is listed here, pick something and do it. Point yourself in the direction of a more exciting sex life and keep moving in that direction.

It is worth it. The payback to you is bigger than the bedroom. Your sex life will be more pleasing and your desire for sex will be greater, and when your sex life heats up, your relationship becomes more compelling. The thoughts about who did the dishes last vanish. It is not because you purposely stop thinking about the household chores—you find yourself relating to your partner in a way that feels bigger and more positive. The pleasure you have in being close to her or him is notably increased. You feel lucky to be alive and together, and the world holds more possibility. You are more forgiving. You feel changed in a way that is positive. You have more extraordinary moments of feeling a sense of oneness, of merging, of melting, of being delighted in the connection you share.

And finally, remember that you are not alone. You are one of millions of intelligent women, many who are hard working and responsible like you, who want to connect sexually in a more powerful way with their mates. Don't buy into the feeling that you are alone, and no one is like you. Yes, you are unique in many ways, but you are not the only one with a desire for more profound sex or a deeper connection. You are not the only one looking for a strong bond and a big love affair. There are 49 million women over the age of 18 in the US with low sexual desire. Ten percent (4.9 million) of these women are bothered that it is low and want to have more sexual desire than they have.[25]

---

25. Shifren, "Sexual Problems," 970-978.

Right now I am picking up my pom-poms, jumping up and down to tell you that you can do this! You can make things more interesting for yourself. You can take action. You will have to show up, speak up, and disclose what works for you. You will probably have to do something new. You can do this.

Appendices

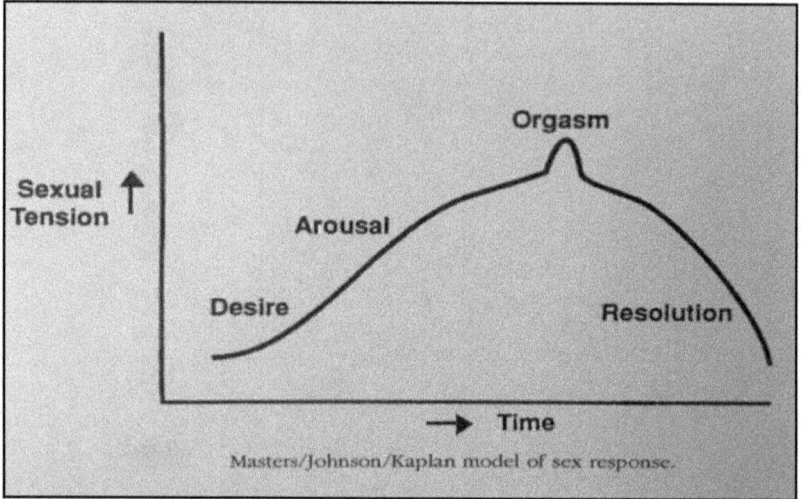

Masters/Johnson/Kaplan model of sex response.

Diagram A.   Female Sexual Response Model - Desire First

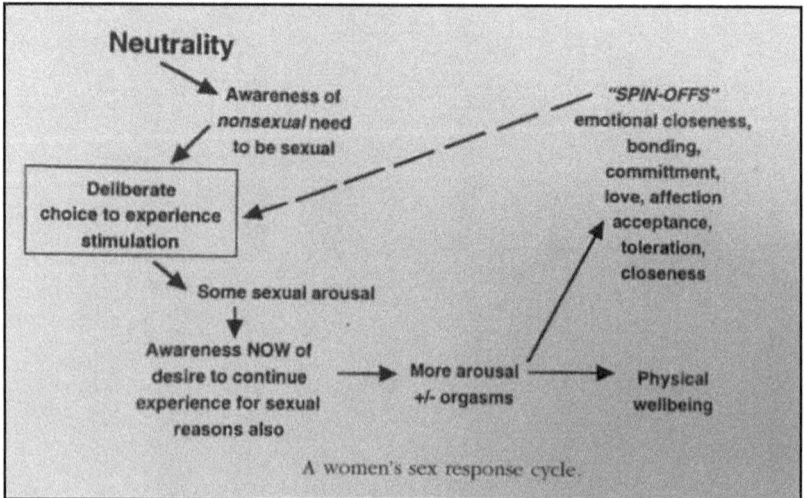

A women's sex response cycle.

Diagram B.   Female Sexual Response Basson Model

Acknowledgments

To the women who shared your stories with me—you are the gems in this book. Although I'm not including your names, I thank you for your profound contribution. You are beauties. Your honest disclosures of the processes that were so personal and life changing have helped lay down a map for other women to use. This map to bedroom treasure would otherwise not exist. It is priceless.

To my husband, Noal Preslar—a hunk of gratitude for your steadfast support over these past seven years with *the book*. Yes, you had quiet eye rolls when I left you downstairs alone, again, for another evening of writing, and yet you delivered dinner to my office with graciousness and a wink. Every time you told me that the world needed what I was writing, you boosted me. Every time you massaged my shoulders you helped this book along. You turned out to be an excellent proofreader, who'd have known? The generous spirit of your love inspires me and I am lucky.

To Carolyn Bond—your positive voice in our first meeting at the coffee shop, and in my first writing attempts, set me up to go. Thank you for that start; you are part of my book.

To Robin Colucci—at our first meeting you said that the editing was going to hurt. You warned that you would take parts out of the book that I liked, possibly my most favorite parts. You said a third or more of what I had written would be removed. You then got the draft and did all of those things. It worked, and I never needed a shot of Lidocaine. Thank you for being the delightful wordsmith that you are.

To Patty and Paul Richards—your regard for the power that sexuality has in awakening us has changed what I know to be possible, both with sex and in being human. This book and my life are more compelling because of you two, and the experiences you have shared with me. If I could give you anything in gratitude it would be permanent access to that luscious Bora Bora lagoon.

To Gretchen Wild—you quickly figured out how I could fit the bike accident story into the introduction. It was an important piece to me and I am grateful.

To our sons, Noah and Spencer, and my stepdaughter Shaney—your natural composure when the subject of my work enters the conversation delights me. You truly rock!

To Fayegail and Sarah—your enthusiastic feedback improved this book and brightened me along the way.

To the *International Society for the Study of Women's Sexual Health* (ISSWSH)—you have provided me a professional home. Since 2005 (when I joined), and even before that, I have had the support of passionate colleagues who care about the same aspects of health and medicine that I care about. These generous ISSWSH colleagues have been available by e-mail and telephone, and have specifically contributed to the sexual success of the women in my practice.

To ALL MY FRIENDS AND FAMILY who I have seen less of socially since 2009, I have missed you too. We will have the grandest shindig when this book gets released.

Here's How You Can Get in Touch with Me

I support women to have a good time in the bedroom. If you want a more personal interaction about how to get going in a good direction, sign up for a *Conversation with Susan* at www.fanningthefemaleflame.com. You can also sign up there for my free electronic newsletter *Sexual Health: News and Views,* and for ongoing educational teleconferences. Finally, if you do turn your bedroom life around, or have already done that, and want to share the details, I would like to hear your story. Email me: susan@ fanningthefemaleflame.com and we will set up a time to connect.

www.ingramcontent.com/pod-product-compliance
Lightning Source LLC
Chambersburg PA
CBHW030021290326
41934CB00005B/435